TREATMENT PLANNING FOR PSYCHOTHERAPISTS

A Practical Guide to Better Outcomes

Second Edition

TREATMENT PLANNING FOR PSYCHOTHERAPISTS

A Practical Guide to Better Outcomes

Second Edition

Richard B. Makover, M.D.
Lecturer in Psychiatry
Yale University School of Medicine
New Haven, Connecticut

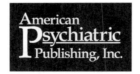

American Psychiatric Publishing, Inc.

Washington, DC
London, England

Note: The author has worked to ensure that all information in this book is accurate at the time of publication and consistent with general psychiatric and medical standards, and that information concerning drug dosages, schedules, and routes of administration is accurate at the time of publication and consistent with standards set by the U.S. Food and Drug Administration and the general medical community. As medical research and practice continue to advance, however, therapeutic standards may change. Moreover, specific situations may require a specific therapeutic response not included in this book. For these reasons and because human and mechanical errors sometimes occur, we recommend that readers follow the advice of physicians directly involved in their care or the care of a member of their family.

Books published by American Psychiatric Publishing, Inc., represent the views and opinions of the individual authors and do not necessarily represent the policies and opinions of APPI or the American Psychiatric Association.

Copyright © 2004 Richard B. Makover, M.D.
ALL RIGHTS RESERVED

Manufactured in the United States of America on acid-free paper
07   06   05   04   03   5   4   3   2   1
Second Edition

Typeset in Adobe's Berling Roman and GillSans

American Psychiatric Publishing, Inc.
1000 Wilson Boulevard
Arlington, VA 22209-3901
www.appi.org

Library of Congress Cataloging-in-Publication Data
Makover, Richard B., 1938–
    Treatment planning for psychotherapists : a practical guide to better
outcomes / Richard B. Makover.—2nd ed.
        p. ; cm.
    Includes bibliographical references and index.
    ISBN 1-58562-148-X (alk. paper)
    1. Psychotherapy. 2. Psychiatry. I. Title.
    [DNLM: 1. Psychotherapy—methods. 2. Planning Techniques.
WM 420 M235t 2003]
RC480.52.M35 2003
616.89′ 1—dc21   2003056061

British Library Cataloguing in Publication Data
A CIP record is available from the British Library.

CONTENTS

PREFACE TO THE SECOND EDITION

I wrote the original version of this book to present a system of treatment planning that would combine a new theoretical structure with practical methods for its clinical use. This new edition builds on that framework with additional emphasis on the formulation as the source of successful planning and on those aspects of the clinical assessment that lead to a useful formulation.

Treatment planning has always been important, but the increasing restrictions of third-party and government sources of financing care continue to create a more pressing need for clear, concise, relevant, and supportable plans. Treatment plans are needed for inpatient care, for discharge to intensive outpatient facilities, and for the initiation and continuation of office-based care. Professional liability issues and the intrusion of regulatory agencies into the therapist-patient relationship also create demands for documentation of specific treatment plans. Of more importance, however, is the way treatment plans help to create more effective care and better outcomes, benefiting both clinicians and their patients.

I am grateful that *Treatment Planning for Psychotherapists* has contributed to this aspect of clinical practice and that it has been useful to mental health professionals in their efforts to meet the need for better-documented treatment planning. I hope this new edition, more concise and with a more practical focus, will continue to be helpful.

PREFACE TO THE
FIRST EDITION

This book is about treatment planning for psychotherapists. It is also about the partnership between us and our patients that will allow us to pursue the best possible outcome for them. Patients come to us in emotional distress and unable to function at their highest level. Planning a course of psychotherapy and implementing that plan can more effectively help them recover from their dysphoric and dysfunctional state.

Because of the wide scope required of any book on so complex a subject as psychotherapy, it is worth noting what this book is *not* about. It is not about how to conduct psychotherapy, although I make liberal use of examples drawn from the way I practice. It is not a survey of the many types of therapy utilized today or an attempt to make any judgment about the efficacy of one therapy over another. It is not about brief therapy, even though treatment planning tends to shorten the length of therapy through an economy of time and effort. It is not about whether insight-expressive therapies are better or worse than directive-supportive therapies. It is neutral in the turf battles among advocates of competing theories. All of these topics have been debated by some of the best theoreticians and practitioners of the last hundred years.

My ideas about treatment planning evolved over the years as I supervised colleagues and trained new psychotherapists. I was impressed with how often a therapy destined for impasse began without identifying the key issues, without an understanding of the crisis that brought the patient in for treatment, and without a clear idea of what might be the best outcome of the work. I came to realize that effective and appropriate treatment planning was a central and persistent challenge, not only for beginning psychotherapists but also for more experienced practitioners.

My supervisees were often puzzled, frustrated, and discouraged when they realized that therapy was no longer working. They were unable to determine the reason and consequently did not know what to do about it. Helping them to reformulate the case and to put together a straightforward treatment plan was often all they needed to get a stalled therapy moving. In peer review discussions, case conferences, and seminars with experienced therapists, I heard many of the same frustrations and complaints. Often a discussion of treatment planning issues—assessment, formulation, treatment contracts, therapy outcomes—helped to clarify and solve the problem.

In putting my ideas about treatment planning into a clinical framework, I have adopted a set of terms—AIM, GOAL, STRATEGY, TACTIC—that are somewhat different from the usual planning terminology (Makover 1992). I have done so in an effort to break away from the more traditional approach. Terminology is, of course, not as important as process, but "new" names may facilitate a fresh look at these important concepts.

At the present writing, treatment planning is emphasized most strongly in the work of multidiscipline treatment teams operating within an institutional environment. I try to offer a system more useful to the individual clinician sitting alone with a patient in an office setting. I hope that those who have struggled with traditional planning will be able to use these concepts in a way that will help them with their clinical work.

This book brings together my own experiences in the practice of psychotherapy with the practical wisdom of many people with whom I have been privileged to work. Writing this book about treatment planning has been educational and gratifying. I hope that it will prove so for the professional reader.

Several friends and colleagues provided support, advice, and assistance. Those I particularly want to acknowledge include Diane Sholomskas, Ph.D., who was a valuable sounding board for my ideas and made useful suggestions about both the substance and the style of the book; Alan Sholomskas, M.D., who provided a thoughtful reading of the completed manuscript; Susan Brown, R.N., M.S.N., whose candid suggestions improved both the content and clarity of my writing; and Daniel Bendor, M.D., who offered many cogent and thought-provoking comments about my ideas.

My wife, Janet Interrante Makover, R.N., M.A., C.N.A.A., offered invaluable advice based on her extensive clinical and administrative experience in this field. I am grateful for her significant contribution to this effort and for her wise counsel.

REFERENCE

Makover RB: Training psychotherapists in hierarchical treatment planning. J Psychother Pract Res 1:337–350, 1992

Chapter 1

HOW IMPORTANT IS TREATMENT PLANNING?

Treatment planning is an organized, conceptual effort to design a program *outlining in advance* what must happen if we are to provide the most effective help for our patients. The plan must make sense to us and represent an effort we feel capable of pursuing to a successful outcome. Of equal importance, the plan must make sense to the patient and allow the patient to use his or her own resources and abilities to achieve the desired results. In today's managed-care environment, the plan must provide measurable outcomes within a reasonable time frame to gain the approval of third-party funding sources. Without a plan, therapy is likely to become diffuse, disorganized, and ineffective; end without resolving the patient's problems; and face reimbursement denial.

An example from psychotherapy supervision shows how unplanned treatment can quickly reach an impasse. Gail, a psychology intern in the hospital's outpatient psychiatry clinic, met with me for weekly supervision and presented a new patient, a man she had seen nine times.

Gary the Gay Gardener

Gary, 37 years old and never married, lived with his lover, Peter, a compulsively promiscuous man who, although apparently committed to Gary, often went out alone to cruise the gay bars and have multiple sexual encounters. Gary was jealous, frightened about AIDS, and angry that he could not control Peter's reckless behavior. He began to experience attacks of panic, and he had brief episodes when he lost his sense of per-

1

sonal identity. His family doctor had given him a tranquilizer, but he hated taking it. Gary worked for a landscape architect and seemed to have a natural gift for design. He was often praised for his ideas, and he had been rewarded with generous salary increases. No one at work knew he was gay; he was not "out of the closet," as he put it. He had not told his family about his sexual orientation, and in fact, only his gay friends knew.

Gail was interested in Gary's secret life. She believed the tension between his gay identity and his straight façade was a deeper reason for his anxiety and depersonalization than the current troubles with his lover. When Gary talked about Peter, she made little response, but when he discussed other areas of his life, especially his work and his family, she actively engaged him in examining these issues. Gary began to talk more about the relatively safe areas Gail responded to and less about the emotional turmoil he felt with Peter. Gail was pleased at the constant supply of new material, but after several weeks she recognized that Gary's anxiety was worse. She asked him to see her psychiatric consultant to get a stronger medication, but he refused, saying he did not want to rely on pills. This answer stymied Gail, and she decided to bring his case to supervision.

Gail had pursued her own treatment objective at the expense of Gary's. His reason for coming into therapy was to resolve the conflicted relationship with his lover. Gail heard this request: she listed it as his "chief complaint." As they began their therapy sessions, however, she shifted her focus to the identity crisis she thought she saw in his concealed sexual preference, and Gary passively accepted her agenda. Perhaps he felt she was the expert and should know what was important. Perhaps the less emotional topic provoked less anxiety in him. Whatever Gary's motives, he did not discuss the problem that was the immediate source of his distress, and his distress did not improve.

How does this treatment impasse reflect a lack of planning? After all, Gail had what she considered a plan: to help Gary "come out of the closet" and thereby resolve his identity conflict, which she believed to be the cause of his symptoms, but her plan had two major flaws. For one, her formulation that Gary's symptoms were a result of his identity crisis ignored the facts revealed in the psychiatric history. For another, Gary and she had not agreed that "coming out" was to be the end point of the therapy. He had not sought help to make that decision; he only wanted Peter to be monogamous. In other words, they had not reached agreement on what they wanted the outcome of therapy to be.

We discussed the flawed formulation and the false agreement in supervision, and Gail made a fresh start with Gary. She asked him whether he would prefer to focus on his social status or instead on the problems with his lover. Gary promptly chose the latter, and Gail agreed to the change. On the basis of her new formulation, that Gary's symptoms arose from the turmoil in his feelings toward Peter, she helped him see that Peter's behavior was too risky and that it demeaned him. He realized he had been putting up with it because of the mistaken notion he was not worth a stable, loving relationship, and he could then give up his "poor me" stance and move on to a better relationship. The issue of his coming out needed no further discussion, and it was dropped. Gail was able to help Gary after she accepted his reasonable request and she directed her skills at the desired outcome. With the therapy refocused, Gary was able to make better use of Gail's help. Improved planning led to a more effective therapy.

A second example raises some different treatment issues. My supervisee, Howard, was a third-year psychiatry resident. With the patient's permission, he had audiotaped some of the sessions.

Hazel the Harried Housewife

Howard described Harriet as a slender, dark-haired woman, age 33, who looked mildly depressed. Her haggard expression confirmed the diffuse anxiety she said was always with her. She entered treatment after her husband remained unemployed six months after losing his job; bills had piled up, and she worried she might lose her home. Her inner turmoil interfered with her sleep and inhibited her appetite. She lost 10 pounds.

Howard decided to hold off offering her medication and to take a supportive approach. He was sympathetic and nonjudgmental and at times offered her some direct advice. For instance, he suggested she turn over all of the bills to her husband, who was not upset by the need to juggle the budget through a lean period. After four weeks of this approach, Hazel's mood was clearly improved. She and her husband both reported that her symptoms diminished, and she even felt well enough to consider stopping the therapy. When her husband returned to work, shortly before her fourth session, her outlook brightened further.

In the meantime, Howard had learned a good deal more about Hazel, including her anxious childhood with an overprotective mother, and he now reformulated the case with a new hypothesis: Perhaps Hazel's childhood experience with her mother sensitized her to the economic stress from her husband's job loss and this sensitivity accounted for her reactive mood change. He pursued this idea through their next two sessions, but in her seventh session Hazel looked worse again. Howard played a portion of the tape:

Hazel: My husband says I'm doing worse lately. He thinks I'm no better now than when I started.
Howard: What do you think?
Hazel: I think he's right. I do. You know, I started to feel better for a while, and I was thinking I should stop therapy, but then a couple

of weeks ago we started talking about my mother and her illness and how hard that was. And now I'm feeling bad again.

Howard: When your husband tells you you're doing worse, what do you think he means?

Hazel: Well, I guess Allen sees me moping around again, and he's worried about me.

Howard: Like your mother used to worry.

Hazel: No, not really. She used to worry about every little thing. Allen isn't like that.

Howard: I wonder if you aren't looking to him for some of the same concern your mother used to give you.

Hazel: Maybe I am. But, you know, now that he's working again, I don't worry so much. I'm sleeping better, and I've gained back the weight I lost. Unfortunately. [She laughs ruefully.] That was the only good thing about how I was feeling before.

Howard: Our time is up for today. We have to stop.

Hazel: All right. I think I'll wait before I make another appointment.

Howard: [Genuinely surprised] Oh? How come?

Hazel: Well, these sessions are pretty expensive. We only get fifty percent back from the insurance. I just can't afford it.

After we listened to the tape, I told Howard what I thought had happened. Hazel presented in a situational crisis that appeared to resolve after a month. No doubt Howard's support was helpful, and when her husband found work, the precipitating stress was relieved. Meanwhile, Howard identified what he thought might be a significant source of her vulnerability. In the last session, he explored one facet of this new theme: whether her husband was infantilizing her now the way her mother had before. Perhaps he was. Hazel's "moping" could indicate this connection was a real one. But Hazel was dropping out, and her decision raised troublesome questions. What happened? Why was she feeling worse after doing so well initially? Why was therapy worth a 50% copayment when they had no current income but not worth it now when they had a paycheck coming in? Why should treatment fail after such a promising beginning?

Was Hazel's early progress only a placebo effect? Was her husband feeling threatened and putting pressure on her to stop? Was she showing resistance? Was the relationship with her mother too painful to deal with? A yes answer to any of these questions places responsibility for the treatment failure on Hazel herself. Before we accept that conclusion, however, we must ask whether the therapist made any contribution to her decision to stop. Did he meet her need for help with a timely, focused, and appropriate intervention?

Up to a point, Hazel's therapy succeeded. She came with a clear request that could be paraphrased as follows: "I am in crisis, and I feel upset.

Please help me get through this bad period in my life. I was doing all right before my husband lost his job, and I hope to do as well afterward. My problem is that I need to find the strength to see it through without falling apart and adding to my family's burden." Howard did in fact meet her request successfully. After four weeks of therapy, her presenting complaints—depressed mood, diffuse anxiety, insomnia, anorexia, weight loss—were gone, and she felt well. She had not asked for more than that, and from a treatment planning perspective, Hazel's decision not to continue makes sense. In the fifth session, however, Howard's enthusiasm influenced his therapeutic judgment. Perhaps he did not realize he had a limited treatment contract with Hazel. When she weathered the situational crisis, she would have been satisfied, but instead of acknowledging their success, Howard began to pursue a new idea as if it had been part of his original plan. Unfortunately he did not tell Hazel about his new approach, about the way it would lengthen her treatment, or about the possibility it would stir up uncomfortable feelings, and he did not secure her agreement to expand the focus of therapy. Over the next two weeks, Hazel became uncomfortable, began "moping around" again, identified the therapy as the new source of her current emotional distress, and decided to stop.

After helping her through the initial crisis, Howard shifted his focus from current stresses to past issues without allowing Hazel to decide whether she wanted to change. What if the proposal to extend the therapy had been handled differently? Imagine that her fourth session included the following dialogue:

> *Hazel:* I've got some good news today. My husband found a job! He starts work next week, and he's even getting a little more money than at the old place.
>
> *Howard:* That *is* good news. You must feel very relieved.
>
> *Hazel:* Oh yes. In fact, I think I'm really better. I don't think I need to come here anymore.
>
> *Howard:* I agree you've now weathered the storm caused by your husband's unemployment. But while we've been talking about your situation, I think I've discovered something about you that makes you more susceptible to the stressful time you went through. I think it has a lot to do with what you told me about your mother and how she used to baby you so much.
>
> *Hazel:* You mean that's why I'm not a confident person?
>
> *Howard:* Yes. Let's explore that idea and see where it leads. If I'm right, you might be able to change how you think about yourself. Then you'd be more resilient in the future when other stressful things come along.
>
> *Hazel:* I guess I could try it for a while. Now that Allen's back at work, it won't be such a strain on our finances. What would I have to do?

> *Howard:* I think we ought to talk some more about the way your mother used to treat you. It might stir up some of your old worries, but I think you can deal with them. And we'd want to look especially at how those old habits are affecting you now.
>
> *Hazel:* I think I'd like to do that. But maybe I should talk to Allen and see what he thinks about it.

Howard would then have proposed a new working agreement with Hazel to pursue his idea about her overdependency, and her last remark, about checking with her husband, might even provide him with a place to start.

THE PSYCHOTHERAPY RELATIONSHIP

In the traditional medical relationship, the doctor prescribes and the patient passively complies. The "good" patient is the one who obediently accepts the recommended treatment. Doctors give expert advice, and patients, as laypersons, are expected to assume doctors know best. In reality, medical patients often behave quite differently, but the expectation of passive compliance remains.

The psychotherapy relationship makes somewhat different demands on our patients. We rely on them to provide us not only with historical information but also with introspective and behavioral data. We want them to be active participants who share in creating their improvement. Although we are expertly trained and experienced, our access to our patients' problems depends in great measure on what they tell us. We therefore expect them to play a dual role. They must be compliant but also collaborative. They must furnish helpful historical information, supply relevant introspective reports, and, if possible, contribute their own treatment ideas. They must be, if not always equal partners, at least significant minority owners of the treatment process, not only active but interactive. These are rigorous demands, but our requirements are equally tough. We must modify the medical practitioner's more authoritarian style to one of greater collaboration. Emphasis on the patient's contribution will oblige us to be more flexible and creative in our expert role. We must be skilled in several treatment modalities, flexible, and willing to restructure the treatment as events determine. Collaboration, dynamic interaction, flexibility—these are difficult requirements, but without them, psychotherapy can fall short of providing its full potential benefit.

HISTORICAL REVIEW

The history of treatment planning in psychiatry is not extensive. Although the literature on psychotherapy is voluminous, published observations about treatment planning are limited, with inpatient treatment planning having thus far received greater attention. Treatment planning for psychiatric inpatients includes both institutional (O'Toole 1982) and multidisciplinary (Galasso 1987; Harper 1989; Kennedy 1992) proposals.

Lewis and Usdin (1982) brought together representative teams from several schools of therapy. Each team outlined treatment planning within its own theoretical framework. Not surprisingly, the behavioral and the somatic treatment schools were able to advance more organized planning schemes than the psychodynamic group. Frances et al. (1984) advocated combining different types of therapy in plans that specify such decisions as the setting, format, duration, and frequency of treatment. They recommended combining somatic, behavioral, and psychodynamic approaches for greater therapeutic benefit.

The "problem-oriented medical record" designed by Weed (1969) quickly became a standard tool for treatment planning across medical disciplines. In psychiatry, however, the simultaneous influence of biological, psychological, and social factors in determining the patient's state of mental health creates difficulties with this approach (Nurcombe 1987). Nurcombe proposed "goal-directed treatment planning," an effort to shift the focus of planning from "problems" to "goals" that can be stated in terms of their measurable "objectives" and can thus be monitored by the therapist as treatment progresses.

Brief therapy methods depend on planning. The work of Davanloo (1980), Malan (1980), Sifneos (1979), and others includes limits on patient selection, on the number of treatment sessions, and on the allowable areas of discussion, as well as other restrictions. Rapid assessment, careful formulation, and a clear understanding with the patient about the desired outcome are all common features of a brief therapy approach. In long-term therapy, these same parameters can make therapy more efficient by minimizing tangential and off-target efforts and by decreasing the unproductive use of therapy time.

The prime objective all therapies share is the desire to ameliorate personal distress and dysfunction, and those who present themselves for treatment expect their distress to be diminished and their function improved. These are reasonable expectations, but how do we know when a course of psychotherapy is effective? Methodological uncertainty about outcome measurement bedevils our efforts to judge the results of our work.

A confounding difficulty with outcome assessment is that almost any psychotherapy system is helpful to some degree. Karasu (1986) described three factors—affective experiencing, cognitive mastery, and behavioral regulation—that operate within all psychotherapies. These nonspecific factors, along with the placebo effect (Garfield and Wolpin 1963), may produce some benefit from any psychotherapy. If the therapist is an empathic, nonjudgmental, benign listener, many patients will benefit, regardless of that listener's theory about what he or she is doing. The efficacy of Karasu's (1986) nonspecific factors alone is difficult to quantify, but it may be significant. Some evidence suggests that many psychotherapy applicants' functioning will improve with little or no formal psychotherapy services. The common observation that patients on a clinic waiting list have improved functioning before being offered formal treatment is an example. The improvement rate can range from 40% (Endicott and Endicott 1963) to 75% (Sloane et al. 1975). If so large a proportion of patients will get better without a formal course of treatment, are we not challenged to provide treatment effective enough to benefit the others?

Patients might mobilize their own resources and use their inner strength and resilience along with our support and encouragement to achieve a favorable outcome from psychotherapy, but sometimes our sincere efforts to help paradoxically block their recovery. Through an imperfect understanding of the patient's needs or persistent misinterpretation of the problem, or simply poor technique, we can divert a patient from the path of healing. A sound treatment plan reduces the chance that our interference in the normal healing process will unintentionally impede progress.

Treatment planning can add to a process that on its own may have a high rate of benefit. Planning seeks to address those situations where the placebo effect and nonspecific factors are insufficient, where the problems are more severe or persistent, or where the patients' own resources are not up to the challenge of solving their problems. It is also a method of structuring the therapeutic effort individually so that it can be understood by the patient and reviewed by the therapist and others on an ongoing basis.

Psychotherapy is an art. Like any art, it requires skilled and competent practitioners. At its best, it is more than a modern version of magical ritual; it is a result of systematic thinking and accumulated experience and is a reliable resource for those who seek our services. It can be taught to new practitioners, and it has a common language through which experienced practitioners can communicate. The art of psychotherapy, in other words, requires rules of procedure and recognizable, repeatable operations that will succeed a high percentage of the time.

ANTIPLANNING BIAS

Nevertheless, the idea of treatment planning offends some who are among the most successful practitioners of psychotherapy. Here, for example, is Yalom (1989) on the subject:

> Indeed, the capacity to tolerate uncertainty is a prerequisite for the profession. Though the public may believe that therapists guide patients systematically and sure-handedly through predictable stages of therapy to a foreknown conclusion, such is rarely the case: instead…therapists frequently wobble, improvise, and grope for direction. The powerful temptation to achieve certainty through embracing an ideological school and a tight therapeutic system is treacherous; such belief may block the uncertain and spontaneous encounter necessary for effective therapy. (p. 13)

Yalom is correct in acknowledging that unexpected developments during therapy are the rule rather than the exception, but his suggestion that planning may obstruct the therapeutic process reflects an unjustified antiplanning bias that remains distressingly prevalent. It rests on a series of often unacknowledged and, in my view, unsupportable beliefs: the belief that human behavior is so mysterious and unpredictable as to render planning useless, the belief that we are too complex to be subject to rational planning, and the belief that the relationship in psychotherapy is *more* important than the therapeutic activity. These ideas contrast with the judgment that psychotherapy is an understandable, teachable treatment process often promoted, sometimes retarded, by the relationship between the parties.

The extensive body of writings from Freud to the present tells us clearly that there are "rules" for psychotherapy, whether it is psychodynamic or behavioral. Generally, these rules apply to the conduct of treatment. They tell the psychoanalyst when to make an interpretation and when to be silent. They tell the behaviorist what to reinforce and what to ignore. There are also rules about what should be treated and by which methods. All of these rules tend to be stated as generalities. Little has been published to specify how an individual patient, sitting across from us in our office, is to be treated.

Like many who were trained when psychoanalysis dominated clinical practice, I was taught that any attempt to structure the treatment or to point it toward a selected outcome would likely damage the therapeutic effort. After all, the argument went, you will not know what the meaningful issues are until, after months or years of listening to your patient, those issues find their way to the surface and reveal themselves in therapy. Anything more than active listening was considered manipulation, or worse, and would adulterate the pure gold of psychoanalytic therapy.

A lot has changed since the 1960s. Daily exposure to the multimedia information network creates informed consumers. Patients expect that their reasonable requests for direct help will receive a fair hearing, and they increasingly seek an active therapy that focuses on their most immediate problems. They more readily accept the idea that some psychological conditions manifest themselves through physical symptoms and that some biological disorders may have important psychological manifestations. Many understand that advances in molecular biology and pharmacology result in more effective medications. We are most often paid for our work by someone other than the patient, and these third-party payers expect us to explain what we are doing, why, and how long it will take. These changes create new and more insistent demands for flexibility, effectiveness, and accountability. The principles and practice of treatment planning provide an effective way to meet these demands.

REFERENCES

Davanloo H: Short-Term Dynamic Psychotherapy. New York, Jason Aronson, 1980

Endicott NA, Endicott J: "Improvement" in untreated psychiatric patients. Arch Gen Psychiatry 9:575–585, 1963

Frances A, Clarkin J, Perry S: Differential Therapeutics in Psychiatry: The Art and Science of Treatment Selection. New York, Brunner/Mazel, 1984

Galasso D: Guidelines for developing multidisciplinary treatment plans. Hosp Community Psychiatry 38:394–397, 1987

Garfield SL, Wolpin M: Expectations regarding psychotherapy. J Nerv Ment Dis 137:353–362, 1963

Harper G: Focal inpatient treatment planning. J Am Acad Child Adolesc Psychiatry 28:31–37, 1989

Karasu TB: The specificity versus nonspecificity dilemma: toward identifying therapeutic change agents. Am J Psychiatry 143:687–695, 1986

Kennedy JA: Fundamentals of Psychiatric Treatment Planning. Washington, DC, American Psychiatric Association, 1992

Lewis JM, Usdin G (eds): Treatment Planning in Psychiatry. Washington, DC, American Psychiatric Association, 1982

Malan D: Individual Psychotherapy and the Science of Psychodynamics. Boston, MA, Butterworth, 1980

Nurcombe B: Diagnostic reasoning and treatment planning: II. Treatment. Austr N Z J Psychiatry 21:483–490, 1987

O'Toole AW (ed): Standards of Psychiatric and Mental Health Nursing Practice. Kansas City, MO, American Nurses Association, 1982

Sifneos P: Short-Term Dynamic Psychotherapy. New York, Plenum, 1979

Sloane RB, Staples FR, Cristol AH, et al: Psychotherapy Versus Behavior Therapy. Cambridge, MA, Harvard University Press, 1975

Weed LL: Medical Records, Medical Education, and Patient Care, Cleveland, OH, Case Western Reserve, 1969

Yalom ID: Love's Executioner and Other Tales of Psychotherapy. New York, Basic Books, 1989

Chapter 2

TREATMENT SELECTION

THREE WAYS OF SELECTING TREATMENT

1. Therapist-Based Treatment

The time-honored way to practice psychotherapy is to become expert in a single methodology and to use it for nearly every patient and for almost every problem the patient presents. Since the mid-twentieth century, one system after another has come into prominence. After World War II, Freud's classical psychoanalysis dominated practice in the United States. Later, other systems rose to challenge its hegemony: the nondirective approach originated by Rogers (1951), Wolpe's (1958) behavior therapy techniques, the transactional analysis of Berne (1961), Beck's (1976) cognitive therapy. More than 400 types of psychotherapy are now available (Bergin and Garfield 1994). As each new methodology developed, its promise of better results encouraged psychotherapists to adopt it, and their investment of time and energy in learning the new system was a strong inducement to use it—if not universally, then wherever possible.

More recently, an exclusive commitment to one school of psychotherapy has given way to a blending of the elements of different methodologies into a self-constructed system. An example would be a therapist whose theoretical framework is psychoanalytic but who interacts with the patient using cognitive interventions. Using an amalgam of theories in an integrated therapy may be effective, but using the *same* amalgamation or integrated system—the therapist's personal school of psychotherapy, so to speak—can be limiting and ineffective.

2. Diagnosis-Based Treatment

Treatment can be selected primarily on the basis of the diagnosis. A clinician might choose a combination of medication and supportive psychotherapy for a man whose condition is diagnosed as "major depression, single episode"; family therapy for an adolescent with "adjustment disorder with disturbance of conduct"; and in vivo desensitization for a woman with "agoraphobia without history of panic disorder." This approach is the decision process used in general medical practice, a model that can be summarized as "assess, diagnose, and treat."

In the mental health field, selecting a treatment on the basis of diagnosis alone is more difficult. Although a task force of the American Psychiatric Association (1989) produced a four-volume compendium of possible treatments for every official diagnostic category, most of the treatments are not specific to the diagnosis, because one therapy approach might be listed under a dozen different diagnostic entities. A more treatment-specific approach, "practice guidelines," is keyed to a single diagnostic entity (Zarin et al. 1993). At this writing, the American Psychiatric Association (2000) has published a compendium of guidelines for entities ranging from delirium and dementias to substance abuse (including nicotine dependence) to anxiety and psychotic disorders. These practice guidelines are part of a growing effort to bring uniformity to the sometimes idiosyncratic field of mental health service delivery. Another type of guideline, the treatment algorithm, uses arrows and choice boxes to diagram treatment decisions, but its strongest proponents acknowledge that the "patient will still need a good doctor" (Jobson 1994, p. 332).

Treatment compendiums, guidelines, and algorithms are not a substitute for individualized treatment planning. Diagnosis-based treatment holds out the promise that the therapist can select the one best treatment for a specifically diagnosed condition, but at the moment it lends itself best to psychopharmacological treatments. Selection of the optimum psychotherapeutic approach is a different matter. Medical diagnosis relies on the "law of parsimony" and seeks a single etiological source for all the patient's symptoms; psychiatric nosology is rarely based on single etiological agents. The majority of our current diagnostic categories depend on description rather than etiology. We match a set of observations to the criteria listed in a diagnostic manual, and these criteria are usually behaviors or subjective reports of internal emotional states. Our diagnoses are seldom based on causative factors, and without causation, diagnosis and treatment cannot be tightly linked.

Multiple determinants operate within and on us. Because we are living organisms with a complex neurophysiology, our mental state is subject to fluctuations in our physical and biochemical systems. At the same time, we are self-aware beings who think and feel in ways that seem independent of our bodies, and we are social beings influenced by interactions with other individuals, with family, and within our community. Each of these systems—biological, psychological, and social—continuously affects us, but in different ways, and each level may be further subdivided. The biological level includes cells, organs, and organ systems; the psychological level includes the individual, the family, and the friendship group; and the social level includes the community, the ethnic group, and the group of national origin. Our knowledge of any one of the levels in this increasingly inclusive hierarchy does not tell us how things work above it or below it. Knowing about the enzymatic activities of a liver cell, for instance, does not tell us how the liver functions. Knowing about the dynamics of a group does not explain all the behavior of one of its individual members. In the same way, these levels of organization can play a role in the patient's psychiatric presentation. A depression may have a cellular basis (low neurotransmitter levels), a family component (a loss within the family), and a social component (ethnic upbringing that imposes a taboo against help seeking). Each level has its own implications for treatment, and the optimum treatment for each may be quite different. "Major depression, single episode" could be treated with medication on the biological level, supportive psychotherapy on the psychological level, and case management intervention on the social level. A man too severely depressed to work, for example, might receive an antidepressant while seeing a therapist weekly for support; the therapist might intervene with his employer to allow him to receive temporary disability benefits.

The diagnosis (and especially, as we shall see later, the formulation that accompanies it) is an important element in the treatment process. If we select treatment solely on the basis of diagnosis, however, we impose a significant limitation on our ability to help our patients.

3. Outcome-Based Treatment

This method of treatment selection looks ahead to the desired result at the end of a projected period of therapy, with the designated outcome based on a variety of factors and determined by a series of decisions. First, we need to identify the problems we will attempt to help the patient solve. That judgment involves not only our recognition of those problems but also the patient's interest in solving them. Second, we need to know what we can realistically accomplish. This conclusion requires not only an appreciation of our own expertise and the techniques we can bring to bear but also our appraisal of the resources the patient can employ. The third step considers the reality factors of time and money, recognizing that a shortage of either will necessarily constrain our efforts. We may have other decisions to make, too. Can the patient be treated in an office setting rather than a hospital? Should we seek help from family members or exclude them? Do we need to collaborate with other providers to use community resources? Our decisions about these multiple factors, taken together, should help us conceptualize the optimum final result of our work with a patient.

STRUCTURE OF OUTCOME-BASED TREATMENT

An outcome-based treatment plan has a four-level structure. First, using our assessment skills to determine the significant problems and the factors bearing on their solution, we must decide which among the various *possible* results of our work with the patient is the single most important and desired outcome of the therapy. I call this desired outcome the AIM. Second, we can envision the enabling conditions. What must happen to bring this outcome about? Stated in specific terms, these enabling conditions will tell us how we can help the patient achieve that one best outcome. These components of the AIM are the GOALS of the therapy. Third, we select which specific therapeutic modalities will best help the patient reach these GOALS. Examples are psychoanalytic psychotherapy, behavior modification, and psychopharmacology. These modalities are STRATEGIES. Fourth, we choose which technical elements to use in pursuit of these STRATEGIES. Examples are interpretations, desensitization, and neuroleptic medications. I call these technical elements TACTICS.

Top-Down Planning

I emphasize that this is a top-down approach. By that I mean that we decide first what we think should be the final outcome of our collaboration with the patient. We next look for the steps that collaboration must develop to arrive at the chosen outcome. The last stage of planning involves choosing the specific means by which we can help our patient take those steps.

By contrast, unplanned or poorly planned treatment takes the opposite path. Its hallmark is the bottom-up approach. The therapist begins

FIGURE 2–1

TREATMENT PLANNING DIAGRAM

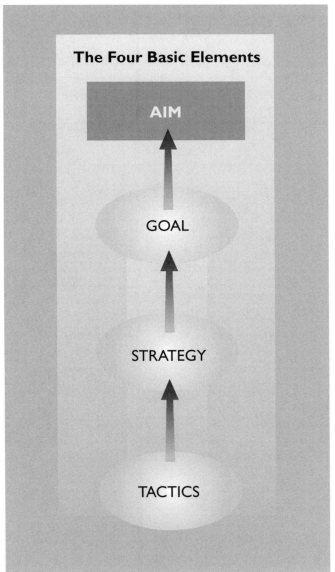

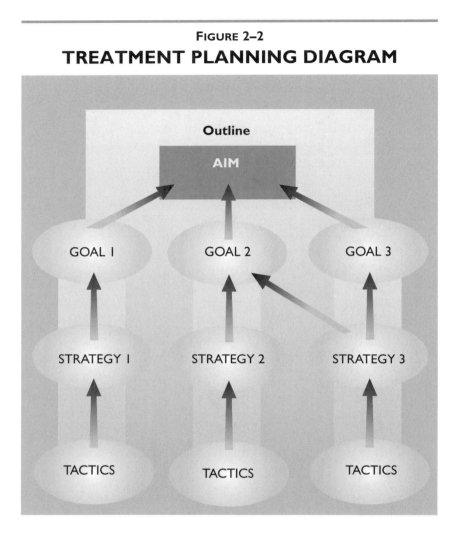

FIGURE 2–2

TREATMENT PLANNING DIAGRAM

with technical maneuvers, through them slides in and out of various therapeutic stances, takes whatever results there are as ex post facto objectives of the work, and accepts the (hopefully favorable) outcome as what was supposed to happen. Bottom-up therapists treat symptoms. They might medicate an anxious mood, attack an ego-dystonic habit with a behavioral paradigm, or offer interpretations as quickly as the patient provides material for the connections. Bottom-up therapists begin treatment somewhere along the expressive-supportive continuum without first deciding what will be the result of operating from that point. They might have some notion of what the therapy should accomplish on the basis of the patient's immediate complaint or of the diagnosis, but the idea is typically vague and abstract—an approximation at best, a guess at worst. Poorly planned bottom-up therapy depends on the placebo effect and on nonspecific factors to heal the patient despite the activity of the therapist.

Well-planned therapy takes a top-down approach from the desired outcome to the means to accomplish it. It thereby attempts to maximize the beneficial effect of the therapist and to add this effect to the nonspecific and placebo factors already at work. Figure 2–1 provides a simple diagrammatic representation of top-down planning. I place the AIM at the top of the hierarchy to indicate it as the first element of the plan. As the arrows in the diagram illustrate, GOALS comprise the AIM; STRATEGY leads to GOALS; TACTICS implement STRATEGIES.

In practice, simple, straight-line plans are uncommon. Most people who come to a psychotherapist for help present more complexity and require branching plans. Figure 2–2 illustrates a plan with three GOALS. One GOAL may require two STRATEGIES. In Figure 2–2, GOAL 2 will be pursued with both STRATEGY 2 and STRATEGY 3. One STRATEGY may serve two GOALS. The figure shows that STRATEGY 3 is directed both at GOAL 2 and GOAL 3.

An Example of Top-Down Planning

To see how these four levels might work in a clinical situation, consider the following fragment of a case history:

Ernest the Edgy Engineer

Ernest was 54 years old, married, and an engineer at a high-technology company; he had been in charge of a small but important project under a government defense contract completed a year earlier. A routine review turned up a minor error, and correcting it reduced the company's profit. He had been a project manager for almost 10 years, and his record had been spotless until the discovery of his "problem." Ernest took the news badly, feeling he had made a serious mistake. He ruminated about it constantly, unable to get his attention onto anything else. Then he had an episode of impotence with his wife and became so preoccupied about that, too, that he was no longer able to function sexually. His wife of 30 years tried to reassure him about both "failures," but he remained unconvinced. At work his brooding became so noticeable that his supervisor asked him to take a leave of absence. His hobbies were gunsmithing and skeet shooting, with occasional hunting trips, and one day his wife found him sitting with a shotgun on his lap and a box of shells open on the table. He explained the incident away, saying he was cleaning the gun for a hunting trip with his son, but his son said they had no such plan. Ernest was a spare, almost gaunt man of precise habits and rigid standards. His health was good, his appetite was unchanged, and his weight was stable. His speech was slow, careful, and circumstantial. He seemed depressed and tense. He denied suicidal ideas. He did not appear to be psychotic.

With an actual patient, of course, we would need much more than this brief vignette before we could arrive at an intelligent treatment plan. Still, even from this little bit of information, we might conclude that Ernest has an obsessional character structure with perfectionistic and overresponsible traits. We can also speculate that he is currently in crisis because he cannot accept any perceived failure without a significant drop in his good opinion of himself, that he has lost confidence and feels ashamed. He may or may not be clinically depressed, and he may be suicidal despite his denial.

We start by asking ourselves: What might be the AIM of his therapy? We can consider three possible outcomes: 1) correction of his characterological impairment, 2) integration of his failures to allow him to resume his life path, or 3) restoration of his ability to work. Notice that these three outcomes differ in their level of complexity and difficulty. Character reconstruction is the broadest and most ambitious AIM. Helping him get past his sense of failure and return to his previous level of function is more modest. The most limited AIM is to get him back to work.

To consider which of these outcomes is best, we take into account that Ernest is a rigid, poorly motivated man in his mid-50s who may not want to devote the time and money to the lengthy treatment we would anticipate if we were to undertake character reconstruction. A little discussion with him confirms our suspicion. He is not interested in long-term therapy; although fearful of more failure, he wants to return to work. Simply getting him back to work, however, might be too modest a result, especially considering the severity of his response to what was, after all, a single, limited failure at his job. He might remain so vulnerable he could easily be upset by another minor setback and once again be unable to function, with a more severe response than before. In addition, this AIM does not address the secondary issue of his sexual "failure." We might suspect his impotence arose at least in part because of worry and shame about his work status, but once it happened, he developed a persistent performance anxiety that could become an ingrained pattern and interfere with his marital relationship. We are left with the middle-level outcome: an effort to help him resume his prior—satisfactory to him—level of function by putting his two failures in perspective: his job setback was not so serious a personal failure that he is unworthy of his professional position; his sexual performance problems are temporary and not

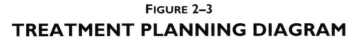

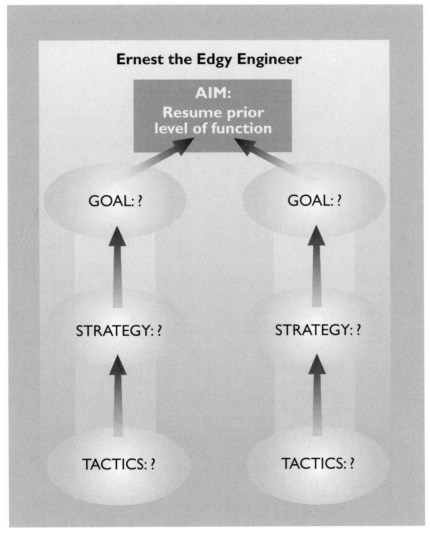

FIGURE 2–3
TREATMENT PLANNING DIAGRAM

Ernest the Edgy Engineer

AIM:
Resume prior
level of function

GOAL: ?   GOAL: ?

STRATEGY: ?   STRATEGY: ?

TACTICS: ?   TACTICS: ?

a reflection on his masculinity. The AIM we have selected can now be placed at the head of a treatment planning diagram (Figure 2–3). Merely as an illustration, I have included space for two tentative GOALS with their possible supportive STRATEGIES and enabling TACTICS. Further planning will address how many GOALS will be needed to achieve the AIM and which STRATEGIES and TACTICS will be required.

We next ask ourselves what has to happen in the course of the therapy for Ernest to resume his prior level of function. One GOAL is to restore his self-image as a competent, reliable professional. A STRATEGY that could lead him to accept this about himself is cognitive therapy. Various cognitive TACTICS might be helpful (e.g., challenging negative overgeneralizations). A second GOAL is to improve his sexual functioning. Here the STRATEGY might be sexual counseling, perhaps including his wife in the sessions. TACTICS could include advising the couple to defer further attempts at intercourse while undertaking a more anxiety-reducing sexual activity, such as sensate-focus exercises. A third GOAL would focus on getting him back to work. Here a case management STRATEGY might come into play. For example, we could, with the patient's permission, contact his supervisor (a TACTIC) and facilitate his reentry. A final GOAL, that of improving his depressed mood, might be deferred until we see the effects of his progress in the other three areas. If we think he is clinically depressed and meets criteria for major depression, we could include this GOAL in our plan. The STRATEGY would be pharmacology. Our TACTIC might be the choice of a selective serotonin reuptake inhibitor on the chance it might ameliorate some of his obsessional symptoms as well, weighing these benefits against the risk that such medication might impair his sexual function. These decisions are placed into our planning diagram (Figure 2–4). The initial diagram listed only two GOALS, but with the planning process completed, we now have four GOALS, each requiring a separate STRATEGY with the necessary TACTICS.

This plan is not the only way to approach Ernest's treatment, and other clinicians might reasonably construct different plans for the same AIM or formulate the case differently to seek a different outcome. For example, one could use Viagra to minimize his erectile dysfunction and help him overcome his performance anxiety. Although there is certainly more than one way to approach a case, however, *effective treatment depends first of all on the clinical judgment about the overall desired outcome of that treatment.*

The top-down plan offers the best chance of asking the right questions, making the right choices, and ultimately having the right answers for our patients. The steps leading up to a proposed treatment plan are critical. They include the assessment of the patient, the formulation of the case, and the construction of the plan itself. Equally important steps then remain and must be taken after the plan is drafted. The plan must be accepted by the patient through a process of negotiation. Therapist and patient must agree on a treatment contract. The completed plan, once under way, must be monitored, often revised, and then finally terminated.

FIGURE 2–4
TREATMENT PLANNING DIAGRAM

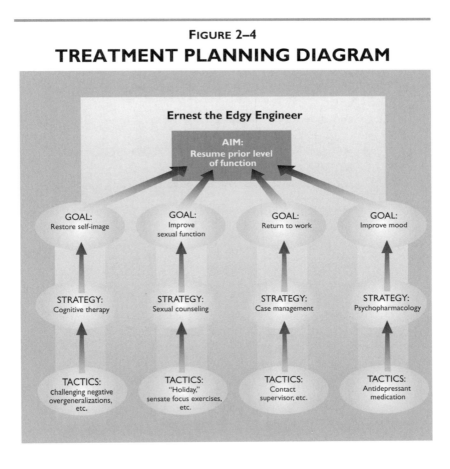

It will be helpful at this point to examine the terminology: AIM, GOAL, STRATEGY, and TACTIC. These terms are discussed in detail in the chapters that follow.

REFERENCES

American Psychiatric Association: Treatments of Psychiatric Disorders: A Task Force Report of the American Psychiatric Association, Vol 1. Washington, DC, American Psychiatric Association, 1989

American Psychiatric Association: Practice Guidelines for the Treatment of Psychiatric Disorders: Compendium 2000. Washington, DC, American Psychiatric Association, 2000

Beck AT: Cognitive Therapy and the Emotional Disorders. New York, International Universities Press, 1976

Bergin AE, Garfield SL (eds): Handbook of Psychotherapy and Behavioral Change. Chichester, England, Wiley, 1994

Berne E: Transactional Analysis in Psychotherapy: A Systematic Individual and Social Psychiatry. New York, Grove, 1961

Jobson KO: Guest editor's commentary: considering treatment algorithms. Psychiatric Annals 24:331–332, 1994

Rogers CR: Client-Centered Therapy: Its Current Practice, Implications and Theory. Boston, MA, Houghton Mifflin, 1951

Wolpe J: Psychotherapy by Reciprocal Inhibition. Stanford, CA, Stanford University Press, 1958

Zarin DA, Pincus HA, McIntyre JS: Practice guidelines. Am J Psychiatry 150: 175–177, 1993

Chapter 3

THE AIM

DEFINITION

The AIM is the single desired outcome of a period of therapy. When we state the AIM of a period of psychotherapy, we expect its achievement to do three things: 1) resolve the distress that brought the patient to us; 2) restore the patient at least to his or her previous level of function, and perhaps even to a higher level; and 3) allow the patient to make further progress, growth, and development. This new term is a departure from current terminology and requires further explanation.

In brief-therapy approaches, one of the critical ideas is the central focus of the work (Ursano and Hales 1986). *Central focus* usually means a single, clearly defined area on which the therapeutic work must concentrate to limit the time course of treatment. Important as this principle is for time-limited therapy, it is a more restricted concept than the AIM, because treatment planning is appropriate for both short and long periods of psychotherapy. A plan may have only a single focus or may require more than one focus to reach the AIM. The concept of a focus has some similarity to what I call a GOAL—that is, it is a well-defined objective of a limited piece of therapeutic work. Each focus (GOAL) may be the central one at a given time, whereas later a different focus (GOAL) becomes central. In short, a central focus of therapeutic effort may be only a part of the overall work that will result in the desired outcome.

Clearly defined outcomes are also a feature of behavior therapy (Taylor et al. 1982). Often they, too, are called GOALS. Behavior therapies are generally based on principles derived from learning theories. The GOALS or objectives are defined operationally—that is, by what the patient will do or not do as a result (e.g., the patient's ability to enter a previously avoided phobic area). Although undoubtedly useful, this idea is also narrower than the AIM. The more inclusive concept usually requires more than one operationally defined objective (GOAL) for its realization.

Table 3–1 lists some representative AIMS with examples of each.

TABLE 3–1.   Examples of AIMS

Category	Example	Desired outcome
Biological	Major depressive episode	Euthymia
Developmental	Transition to old age	Eriksonian integrity
Situational	Unexpected job loss	Crisis resolution
Existential	Prolonged bereavement	Acceptance
Psychodynamic	Oedipal object choices	Mature relationship

The following five clinical examples illustrate the AIMS listed in the table.

EXAMPLE 1: BIOLOGICAL

A major depressive episode is a typical example.

Derek the Depressed Dentist

Derek, a 33-year-old dentist who was married and the father of 10-year-old twin girls, had a successful practice and was active in his community, serving on the board of a local food bank charity. He owned a custom-built house, a vacation home on an upstate lake, three cars, and two boats. Sometime during the winter, he began to awaken early in the morning feeling terrible and was unable to get back to sleep. His appetite declined, and he lost 10 pounds. Gradually he noticed he had less energy to pursue his interests and, as time went on, less interest in trying to do so. He withdrew from his family, found excuses not to honor his community commitments, and felt hopeless about his life and his inability to function. Although he found his professional work burdensome and had difficulty leaving his house in the morning to go to the office, he managed to keep up his practice. His mood lifted a bit by evening, but he felt low again the next morning. Vague thoughts of suicide entered his mind. When he looked for reasons not to give in to them, only his concern for his family made him reject the thoughts. Derek had never experienced anything like this persistently discouraged mood. He went to his family doctor in hopes of being told there was something physically wrong with

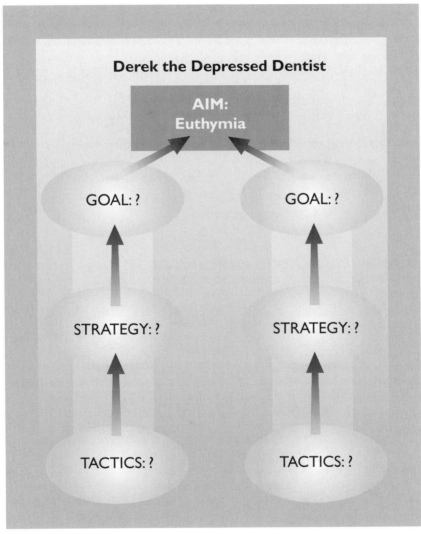

FIGURE 3–1

TREATMENT PLANNING DIAGRAM

Derek the Depressed Dentist

AIM:
Euthymia

GOAL: ?   GOAL: ?

STRATEGY: ?   STRATEGY: ?

TACTICS: ?   TACTICS: ?

him, something for which he could take some pills and be rid of it. The doctor examined him, ran some tests, and then told him he was suffering from "depression."

Although Derek's disorder has a biological basis, we should not exclude psychological and social factors, such as the emotional strength that allowed him to keep up his dental practice in the face of disabling symptoms and the additional stress of social pressures when he could not continue his community service activities. We must include all relevant factors in our plan.

A wealth of evidence suggests that a temporary deficiency of central nervous system neurotransmitters underlies some of the signs and symptoms of a depressive disorder. A return to normal neurotransmitter levels seems to parallel improvement. A normal mood, euthymia, is the desired outcome—the AIM—when we treat someone with clinical depression, and we can enter this AIM at the top of a treatment planning diagram (Figure 3–1).

Note that at this point we have not said what it would take to bring about this change or what we propose to do to make it happen. The AIM sets our sights on a destination toward which we want the therapy to travel. The road we select, how we proceed down it, and what signposts we look for along the way will depend on our assessment of the patient and our subsequent decisions.

EXAMPLE 2: DEVELOPMENTAL

Developmental issues figure prominently in the lives of people who seek psychotherapy. They arise from transitional points in childhood and adult maturation. Examples include going away to school or military service, getting married or becoming a parent for the first time, adjusting to retirement, and aging. Times of change and uncertainty are naturally stressful to all of us, but some people struggle more in getting through them, and some get stuck. The stress associated with these difficult transitions can precipitate a request for psychotherapy.

Erikson (1950) described eight of these "stages of man" and paired success and failure for each, as shown in Table 3–2.

Erikson thought successful resolution of the first stage, in infancy, results in a trusting attitude toward the world but that lack of resolution results in "basic mistrust" that can influence future expectations. He suggested that at the other end of life, normal development gives individuals a sense of "ego integrity" that helps them face their approaching death with equanimity. A failure to achieve this stage leaves the person in a state of despair, bitterly resentful that life has been too short.

TABLE 3–2. Erikson's "stages of man"

Stage	Eriksonian dichotomy	Time period
1	Trust versus mistrust	Postnatal
2	Autonomy versus shame and doubt	Infancy
3	Initiative versus guilt	Toddler
4	Industry versus inferiority	Latency
5	Identity versus role diffusion	Adolescence
6	Intimacy versus isolation	Young adult
7	Generativity versus stagnation	Adulthood
8	Integrity versus disgust and despair	Maturity

Source. Adapted from Erikson 1950.

Dorothy the Despairing Dowager

Dorothy was 67 years old and had never married. Her career as an accountant kept her busy and satisfied, and when she decided to retire at age 65, because her Social Security and retirement benefits would make an earned income unnecessary, financial logic had prevailed over her desire to keep busy. Now, two years later, she was bored and disillusioned. Her younger sister was happily involved in raising four daughters, and she envied her sister's success as a mother. On a deeper level, she resented that her sister, now in her late 40s, could look forward to so many more years than she could expect for herself. Although she had no significant health problems, she brooded over the minor aches and ailments that told her she was growing older. Many times she would sit alone in her darkened bedroom and weep for herself and her "wasted" life. When she visited her sister or played a game of bridge with friends, she put on what she thought was a cheerful façade, but despite her effort, others recognized in her sarcastic jokes and gloomy predictions about current events that she was not the Dorothy they had known. Her oldest friend visited her from another state and pointed out this change to her. She was then able to tell her friend she was in a state of despair and had no idea what to do about it.

An older woman who comes to therapy feeling overwhelmed by this sense of despair may not be clinically depressed, as she might first appear. Dorothy shows none of the "neurovegetative signs" that plagued Derek: Her sleep, appetite, and energy are unaffected; she does not feel hopeless or have suicidal thoughts. She is caught in the grip of a transitional challenge, and the AIM, the single most inclusive and best outcome, would be to help her achieve an Eriksonian kind of integrity (Figure 3–2).

FIGURE 3–2
TREATMENT PLANNING DIAGRAM

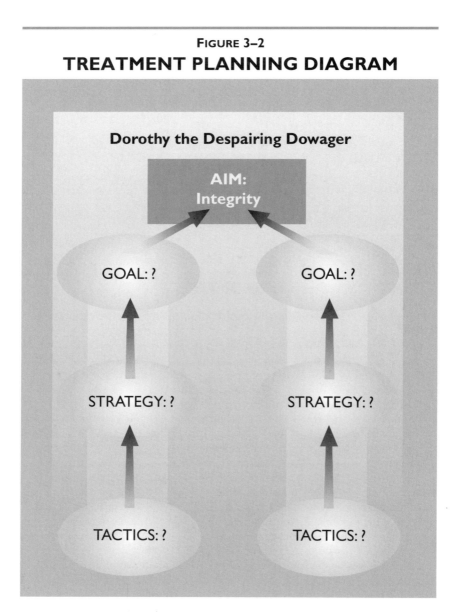

FIGURE 3–2

EXAMPLE 3: SITUATIONAL

Situational problems often initiate a request for psychotherapy. The individual's ordinary level of function may be less than optimal, yet if the environment is stable, he or she can tolerate it. Let some additional stress enter the picture, even one that might in itself be rather mild, however, and it can become the proverbial straw that breaks the camel's back.

Ulysses the Unemployed Undertaker

Ulysses, a 24-year-old single man, lived at home with his parents. He had worked for five years for a local funeral home, learning on the job, and the funeral director, a friend of his parents, had taken an interest in him. Ulysses thought he would move up in the business, perhaps one day becoming a director himself. Unfortunately, the funeral director had a son as well. When his own boy was ready to enter the workforce, the director decided to bring him into the business, and he told Ulysses he would have to let him go because he could train only one person at a time. Ulysses was shocked by this unexpected blow. He had dreamed of saving money, moving out of his parents' home into an apartment, expanding his social life, and possibly even getting married. Instead his future was now uncertain. He became diffusely uncomfortable, with a sense of foreboding and apprehension; brooded about his problems; and had trouble falling asleep. Never comfortable in social situations, he had gained confidence from his work status and could more easily converse and joke with others, but now he became reclusive, embarrassed that he was unemployed and unwilling to face people who might ask him about his work. His parents' efforts to cheer him up and to encourage him to go out made no difference. He had been a social drinker, but now he began taking small drinks throughout the day and as a nightcap. He filed an unemployment claim but made only token efforts to find new work.

The unexpected stress of being laid off has thrown Ulysses into turmoil. Anxiety has increased, sleep has become disturbed, and drinking has increased in a self-medicating effort. Situational problems often present in this manner. New symptoms appear or existing symptoms worsen, and the individual's level of distress impairs function. The lower level of function further deepens the crisis and leads to even less effective coping. Yet once the situation that brought the additional stress disappears, so can the symptoms. It is as if the individual can deal with only so many "units" of stress at one time. Increase those units, and adjustment declines. Reduce them, and it rises again.

Given these parameters, the single best overall outcome (the AIM) would be resolution of the crisis. Ulysses might be expected to resume at least his prior level of function if he could find new employment, especially if it was something he was again proud to do. This rather concrete outcome might well resolve the crisis (Figure 3–3).

FIGURE 3–3
TREATMENT PLANNING DIAGRAM

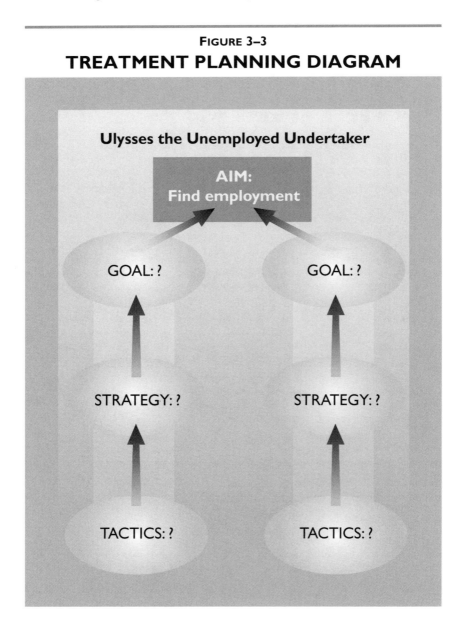

EXAMPLE 4: EXISTENTIAL

Existential problems arise from the usual and expected—one could almost say "normal"—stresses of the human condition. Time marches on. Life is short. Death and taxes…and so on. We embody these profound issues in trite aphorisms, yet they play a significant role in our emotional life. Although usually in the background of our thoughts, they can at times become so overwhelming as to impair function. The death of a spouse is one such existential ordeal. It confronts the survivor with the inevitable impermanence of close relationships. Although its stress is severe, most meet the challenge and with time can move ahead with their lives. Wendy is an example of someone who could not.

Wendy the Weeping Widow

Wendy, 45 years old, had been happily married until 3 years earlier when she and her husband, Walter, were playing golf on a pleasant Sunday afternoon, and he suddenly fell unconscious. Wendy stood by helplessly as others dashed back to the clubhouse to call an ambulance, but Walter died within minutes from what she later learned was a massive heart attack. She and Walter had not had children, and she used to say Walter was her whole life. Wendy went through the funeral in a state of numb disbelief. At times she felt as if she was watching herself perform the necessary actions. In the weeks after the funeral, she seemed to regain her old self, but soon she was able to think of little else except her loss. Sometimes she thought she could see Walter's face, and there were even a few times when she felt he had come into the room. Once or twice she was almost sure she heard his voice. Wendy withdrew from her old, active social life and discouraged her friends from coming to see her. She lost herself in reading romance novels while she solaced herself with sweets and gained weight. Escaping into sleep, too, she went to bed early and slept until noon. These habits occupied her for 3 years after Walter died.

Although grief is a normal and indeed restorative response to loss, the process of grieving can become so prolonged as to prevent the individual from accepting the world without the loved one. The best outcome of therapy (the AIM) for such a person is to come to terms with, to accept, the loss and to move on with life. We can place *acceptance* at the top of our planning diagram to represent this AIM (Figure 3–4).

FIGURE 3–4

TREATMENT PLANNING DIAGRAM

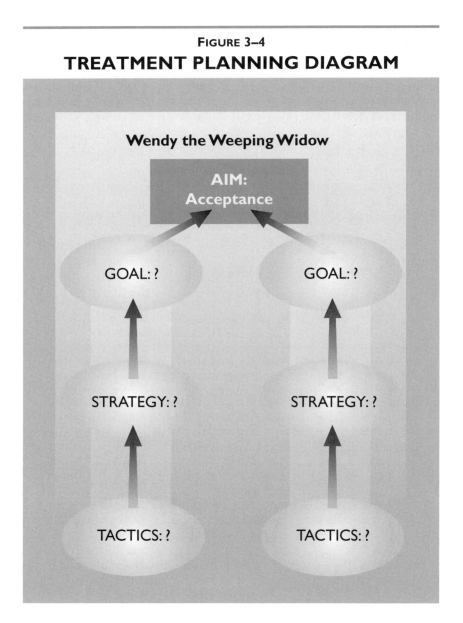

EXAMPLE 5: PSYCHODYNAMIC

Psychodynamic issues are always present in our lives, out of awareness and undoubtedly more potent as a result. These psychological forces and counterforces act within us and on us, shaping our behavior. An example of the Freudian concept of oedipal object choice is the case of Pablo.

Pablo the Panicked Painter

Pablo, a 37-year-old painter of portraits and landscapes, liked to think of himself as a free spirit. He had never married, but he pursued women relentlessly. Models, fellow artists, patrons, casual pickups—Pablo liked to say that women were always available. He was especially interested in married women and preferred having affairs with them because he considered them to be safe. Since they were already married, he need not worry about their expecting a proposal from him. Each conquest was followed by a period of intense involvement, lasting from a few weeks to several months, and then he would grow bored and restless, break off the relationship, and search for a new one. Pablo was an only child. His father, a wealthy and powerful businessman with political connections, urged him to pursue sports and expected him to come into the family business after college. When Pablo persisted in his artistic interests, his father became critical and then would have nothing further to do with him. His mother appreciated his talent, however, and she encouraged him to develop it and to pursue a career in art. Pablo remained close to her, calling her his biggest supporter and his fairest critic. Her only criticism was reflected in her wish that he would marry and settle down.

Over the years Pablo maintained an on-again-off-again relationship with Phyllis, one of his art-school instructors. She was somewhat older, and he thought she was especially attractive. Their earlier sexual relationship had now become a steady friendship, and Pablo liked to see her when he was between affairs, but Phyllis surprised him one day by telling him she had decided to end their friendship. Although he pressed her for reasons, she refused to explain herself beyond commenting that he ought to figure it out for himself. After Phyllis's declaration, Pablo tried to shake off his anger and move on with his life. He increased his pursuit of other women with one-night stands and brief liaisons and sometimes would see two women a night. Despite this frenetic dating, he felt lonely and unhappy. Always diligent in his work, now for the first time he had difficulty concentrating, and his progress on several commissioned works slowed. Even his mother noticed something was wrong, and she urged him to "get some professional help."

Pablo's oedipal conflict fuels his inability to turn his superficial, transitory relationships into a single permanent one. It is as though he was stuck in midadolescence, measuring his social success by the "notches on his gun belt." The AIM of our work with Pablo would be to help him achieve a mature love relationship (Figure 3–5).

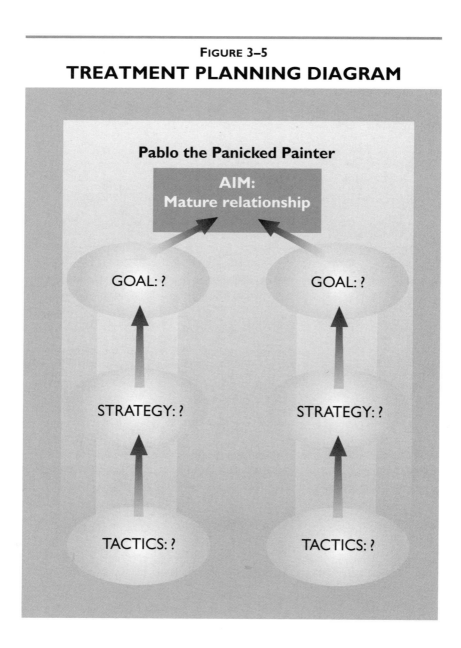

FIGURE 3–5

TREATMENT PLANNING DIAGRAM

Pablo the Panicked Painter

AIM:
Mature relationship

GOAL: ?

GOAL: ?

STRATEGY: ?

STRATEGY: ?

TACTICS: ?

TACTICS: ?

DISCUSSION OF THE AIM

As we can see by these examples, the single desired outcome—the AIM—will usually be the successful resolution of one broad problem area and has four requirements:

1. The AIM should be inclusive—that is, it should bring together all of the identified complaints under one encompassing idea, following the "law of parsimony" to achieve the most economical statement of what the patient will accomplish if therapy succeeds.
2. The AIM should be specific—that is, it should delineate the desired outcome in the most concrete and relevant fashion possible. A non-specific AIM might be *increased self-esteem*, a vague term, difficult to define. It is a part of so many patient presentations as to be almost meaningless and so general as to resist successful achievement.
3. The AIM should be realistic—that is, it should be achievable by that particular patient. This judgment requires an accurate assessment of the patient's strengths, suitability for the contemplated therapy, and ability to benefit from it. The judgment might rest on both intrinsic factors (such as intelligence and motivation) and on extrinsic factors (such as health insurance coverage or prior experience with psychotherapy).
4. Achieving the AIM should require an economy of effort—that is, it should entail no more than what the patient wants from therapy and what the therapist is able to provide. The AIM should be the center of the therapeutic contract, the agreement between patient and therapist as to what they will try to do together.

Each period of therapy should have only one AIM. As the work progresses, the patient may stray from the agreed path, sometimes—but not always—as a resistance. The alert therapist will try to deal with this divergence at an early moment. Equally, the therapist may become interested in new treatment directions, tempting her or him to pursue material unrelated to the agreed objective. If the other material is compelling and relevant, and if the original AIM has been achieved, the therapeutic agreement can be renegotiated. Patient and therapist can then begin a new period of therapeutic work with a new AIM, but until then, fidelity to the agreed objective will best serve the patient's interest.

Therapists who are unfamiliar with the planning process may have difficulty moving from the theoretical concept of an AIM to the practical definition of an overall outcome. Part of the difficulty may be the novelty of expecting a definite end point, especially one that can be discussed in advance with the patient. To facilitate this effort, one might ask: What would need to happen for this therapy to be entirely successful? If this patient were to achieve the best possible recovery from the present difficulties, what would his or her life be like?

After deciding on the AIM, planning then moves to the next level—selection of GOALS.

REFERENCES

Erikson EH: Childhood and Society. New York, WW Norton, 1950

Taylor CB, Liberman RP, Agras WS, et al: Treatment evaluation and behavior therapy, in Treatment Planning in Psychiatry. Edited by Lewis JM, Usdin G. Washington, DC, American Psychiatric Association, 1982, pp 151–224

Ursano RJ, Hales RE: A review of brief individual psychotherapies. Am J Psychiatry 143:1507–1517, 1986

Chapter 4

GOALS

DEFINITION

A GOAL is one of the *subsidiary* objectives of therapeutic work and therefore a component of the AIM. The realization of that single desired outcome, in other words, first requires the achievement of one or more GOALS. Usually two to four GOALS are needed, each addressing a portion of the overall task.

If the AIM translates into only one GOAL, then the outcome of therapy equates with the attainment of one specific and measurable objective. In this instance we "operationalize" the AIM and translate it from an expected result into a statement of what that result would comprise. For example, suppose our encounter with Ernest the Edgy Engineer[1] was in the capacity of a counselor in his company's employee assistance program and we were allowed no more than three visits in-house before we made a referral to an outside provider. The AIM of our brief therapy would probably be to help him return to work, using only one of the four GOALS we chose in pursuit of the more ambitious AIM of restoring him to his previous level of function.

More than four GOALS are also possible, but they should not be needlessly multiplied, because the therapy then tends to become overly complex and cumbersome. A closer look will often reveal that some GOALS are diffuse, poorly defined, too concrete, or inaccurate. It is also possible, when there are multiple GOALS, that two or more may be restated as one. In Ernest's case, for example, we might have chosen two additional

---

[1]See case vignette, Chapter 2, pages 19–20.

GOALS: 1) increase his confidence and 2) restore his professional pride. Adding these two to the four original GOALS—restoring his self-image, helping him return to work, improving his sexual function, and improving his mood—would give us six. We could think about a seventh GOAL as well if we defined it as his being able to accept his mistake as understandable human fallibility. "Improved sexual function," however, will likely have a beneficial effect on his confidence, and "restoring his professional pride" requires that he come to terms with his mistake and move on in his career. Confidence and professional pride are qualities contained within the GOAL of restoring his self-image, and this one GOAL can serve in place of the other two. "Accepting his mistake" is also a necessary step in restoring his self-image, and this seventh objective is included in the GOAL of restoring his self-image as well. Three of the GOALS on this expanded list, then, are unnecessary and are already included in one of the original four.

A GOAL must be stated in operational terms. To do so requires us to specify observable, measurable phenomena, such as particular behaviors, that we can describe and document. Not only is this requirement useful in conducting the therapy, but it is often needed to respond to the demands of case managers and other reviewers. In the case of Ernest, one of the GOALS was *return to work*. More abstract terms such as *employability* or *work readiness* would be less helpful because we would not know whether Ernest was again employable or even whether he were really ready for work until he successfully returned to work. Another way we might define this GOAL is *decrease work anxiety*. This definition would make it hard to gauge our progress. How is work anxiety measured? We want to be able to know when we have reached the end point of this aspect of the therapy. By stating the GOAL as *return to work*, we can know exactly when Ernest succeeds at it.

Sometimes it is difficult to translate an AIM into the components necessary to bring it about. When this happens, it may be helpful to ask, what different things have to happen for the patient to achieve the AIM of the therapy? For Ernest, once we select as the AIM that he resume his prior level of function, it is clear that to do so he needs to reverse the factors that had lowered it. His history suggests four such factors: he was out of work, his sexual competence had diminished, his mood was low, and his self-image was poor. From that point in the analysis, GOALS were easily defined by describing the reverse of each factor.

Although achieving the AIM requires that all of the GOALS must be met, they do not all need to be reached simultaneously. It may make sense to complete one effort before shifting focus to another. The first GOAL may facilitate work on the second. Ernest may, for example, need to respond to the antidepressant medication before he can mobilize the energy and interest to improve his sexual function. The successful accomplishment of one effort may strengthen the patient's confidence and provide help with the next effort. Ernest might feel better enough about himself when his sexual function improves to reexamine his professional activities with a kinder eye.

The general principle, then, in defining and selecting GOALS is that each should be as inclusive as possible, as long as it is defined in concrete, operational terms.

EXAMPLE 1: DEREK THE DEPRESSED DENTIST

Derek is the 33-year-old successful professional, family man, and community activist who slipped gradually into a hopeless, withdrawn mood.[2] We based our AIM, euthymia, on the premise that his depression reflected a biological disorder. One of our GOALS, therefore, would be to correct the underlying biochemical abnormality that we can summarize (in an oversimplification) as low neurotransmitter levels. We need an operational statement of this GOAL. *Raise neurotransmitter levels to normal* is such a statement, but it would be unrealistic because at present, we cannot measure brain neurotransmitter levels in the clinical laboratory. We can quantify the symptoms of his depression by asking Derek to complete one of the available rating scales, such as the Hamilton Rating Scale for Depression (Hamilton 1960), and then state the GOAL as a lower number score on the Hamilton scale. Suppose, however, that we do not want to present Derek with a series of written tests. Perhaps it would make him feel like an object to be studied rather than a fellow human being and thereby damage the therapy relationship. Another way to define this GOAL operationally would be to follow his presenting symptoms as revealed in the mental status examination: sleep disturbance, diurnal mood variation, anorexia, low energy, impaired concentration, and suicidal ideation. The GOAL can then be stated as *eliminate depressive symptoms*.

We might now ask whether eliminating the depressive symptoms is not the same as our AIM of euthymia. It is not. We have not included in

---

[2]See case vignette, Chapter 3, pages 26–27.

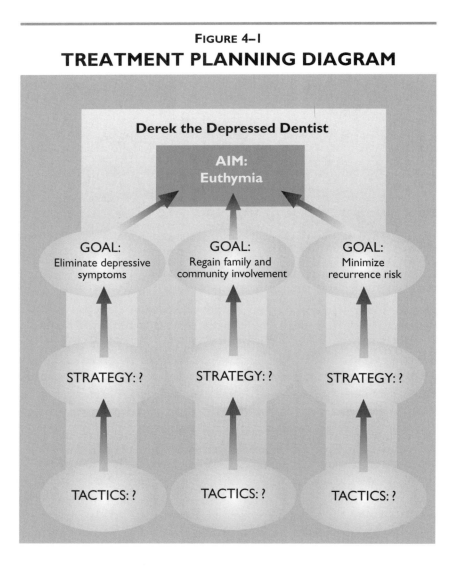

FIGURE 4–1
TREATMENT PLANNING DIAGRAM

Derek the Depressed Dentist

AIM:
Euthymia

GOAL:
Eliminate depressive
symptoms

GOAL:
Regain family and
community involvement

GOAL:
Minimize
recurrence risk

STRATEGY: ?

STRATEGY: ?

STRATEGY: ?

TACTICS: ?

TACTICS: ?

TACTICS: ?

our list of symptoms the more global signs of the depression: the change in his overall level of function and the hopeless mood itself. Remember that he withdrew from family and friends and avoided his community activities, previously a significant source of satisfaction for him. He also struggled to maintain his dental practice. The neurovegetative symptoms alone do not reflect these broader difficulties. His overall mood will have to return to his premorbid, more optimistic outlook before he can be said to be euthymic.

We will need a second GOAL to address the interpersonal and social difficulties. It might be phrased "regain family and community involvement."

A final GOAL to consider would be based on our recognition that major depression has a tendency to recur. Although this appears to be Derek's first episode, he will be at higher risk for a second depression. If we wanted him to continue taking the medication for perhaps another year after he recovers, we would add a GOAL of *minimize recurrence risk*.

Our GOALS for Derek (Figure 4–1) are 1) eliminate depressive symptoms, 2) regain family and community involvement, and 3) minimize recurrence risk.

EXAMPLE 2: DOROTHY THE DESPAIRING DOWAGER

Dorothy is the unmarried accountant who finds herself bitter and disheartened in retirement.[3] The AIM we chose, a sense of integrity about her life, was based on an appreciation of her challenge at the final stage of Eriksonian development. Now we must translate the abstract idea of integrity into operational terms that would be our road map for helping her get there. Her history points us toward two central problems. First, Dorothy's sense of a wasted life is at least partly derived from not having children. She envies her younger sister, whose four daughters seem to give her life a purpose and meaning that Dorothy's lacks. Well past childbearing age and too old to adopt, Dorothy confronts the unpleasant fact that her opportunity for motherhood is irretrievably lost. Second, she is no longer engaged in her life's most important activity, her work as an accountant. That source of pride and gratification is now only a memory, and nothing is available to take its place. In response to these frustrations, she is pessimistic about her current stage of life. She realizes she has come much farther than she has to go, that she is just waiting to die. Her overconcern with minor physical complaints, a kind of hypochondriacal anxiety, reflects this pessimism.

Erikson defined *ego integrity* in broad cultural terms, reflecting the individual's appreciation of his or her place in history and in the lives of others (Erikson 1950). Our AIM for Dorothy might be less ambitious. Perhaps we can help her see that these are also years of opportunity. We

---

[3]See case vignette, Chapter 3, page 29.

FIGURE 4–2

TREATMENT PLANNING DIAGRAM

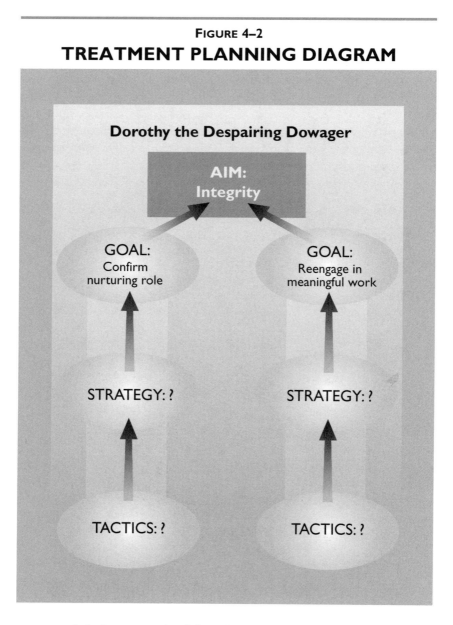

can try to help her accept her life as the best she could have lived, to view the choices she made without 20/20 hindsight, and to view this stage of her life as the natural culmination of her earlier achievements and a worthwhile period of living.

On the basis of her history, the two GOALS that could help Dorothy work toward this outcome would address the issues of childlessness and of the loss of meaningful work. For the first, we could help her redefine the issue of childlessness by looking at others whom she had nurtured, such as younger colleagues to whom she was a mentor. She might find expression for her maternal feelings through activities with children who are not hers; perhaps she could become more involved in the care and up-bringing of her sister's children. We would call this GOAL *nurturance.* For the second GOAL, we would look for something in her current life that would be equivalent to the meaningful work she pursued before retire-ment. She might, for example, volunteer as a consultant to those trying to start a new business or do taxes for other retired people. She might think of other ways to fulfill both her need for nurturance and her need for meaningful work; of course, the choice would be hers. Perhaps all we are saying here is that Dorothy needs to fulfill Freud's definition of men-tal health: to love and to work.

These GOALS do not in themselves constitute the integrity that is the AIM of our work with Dorothy. What they could provide is a basis for her to accept her present stage of life as satisfactory, one with which she can come to terms and appreciate for its own sake.

These GOALS (Figure 4–2) would be to 1) confirm her nurturing role and 2) reengage in meaningful work.

EXAMPLE 3: ULYSSES THE UNEMPLOYED UNDERTAKER

Ulysses was apprenticed in a funeral home but felt devastated when he was supplanted by the director's son. His latent social phobia worsened, and he began drinking too much.[4] Our hope of getting him through this crisis lay in our AIM of getting him back into the workforce. What keeps Ulysses from returning to the work? His anxiety symptoms, for which he is self-medicating with alcohol, are certainly a problem, and so is his stalled effort at job hunting. He is using his unemployment compensation to spare him the stress of seeking a new position. His avoidance of social situations contributes to his paralyzing sense of inadequacy and confirms his belief that he cannot enter a work situation. These identified prob-lems lead to the GOALS we would propose for him. Relief from anxiety symptoms without alcohol is one necessary step. A second is to resume

---

[4]See case vignette, Chapter 3, page 31.

his social activity. The third is an active and serious effort to find another job.

Another consideration is whether a latent alcohol addiction was activated by the stress of being terminated and could persist even if that stress were removed by a new job. If we conclude his drinking was not merely self-medication but was in fact early alcohol abuse, we will need to add a fourth GOAL—*abstinence*.

For the present, then, our GOALS (Figure 4–3) would be 1) symptom relief, 2) social reengagement, and 3) effective job seeking.

FIGURE 4–3
TREATMENT PLANNING DIAGRAM

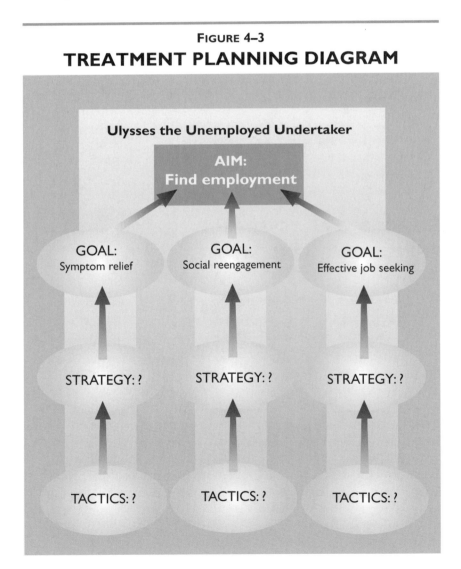

Ulysses the Unemployed Undertaker

AIM:
Find employment

GOAL:
Symptom relief

GOAL:
Social reengagement

GOAL:
Effective job seeking

STRATEGY: ?

STRATEGY: ?

STRATEGY: ?

TACTICS: ?

TACTICS: ?

TACTICS: ?

EXAMPLE 4: WENDY THE WEEPING WIDOW

Wendy, whose husband died suddenly and dramatically on the golf course, has been unable to accept her loss and, at age 45, has retreated into daydreaming and sleep.[5] We defined this problem in existential terms and set her acceptance of her husband's death as the AIM of our therapy. In devising GOALS for her, we must pay attention not only to her ineffective grieving process but to the unhealthy consequences of her bereavement: social withdrawal, overeating, oversleeping, and escape into romance literature. The gratifications gained through these symptomatic behaviors appear to outweigh the emotional cost of her withdrawal. One of our GOALS should be to facilitate (actually to restart) the grieving process. On the basis of the scanty information we have so far, we can assume that no hidden pathology—a latent psychosis, for instance, instead of the mild dissociative symptoms—prevents her from normal mourning and that once she allows herself to begin, she will complete the process. A second GOAL must address the negative symptoms. We can state this GOAL as *resumption of former lifestyle*, to the extent she can resume it without her husband. We would expect her, for example, to begin to re-involve herself with friends, including playing golf again, instead of spending her time in bed. What about another marriage? The void in Wendy's life might be filled if she found another partner to share it with, but we would not want to set this possibility as a GOAL of psychotherapy. At this point, Wendy cannot consider a new attachment because she is struggling to disengage her feelings from the relationship with Walter. Successful mourning is a process extending over at least two years, longer than Wendy may be in therapy, and many therapists would feel uncomfortable with the role of matchmaker. Remarriage would be an inappropriate GOAL for us to consider for Wendy.

The two GOALS (Figure 4–4) we might propose for Wendy, then, are 1) reactivation of the mourning process and 2) resumption of prior active involvements with others.

---

[5]See case vignette, Chapter 3, page 33.

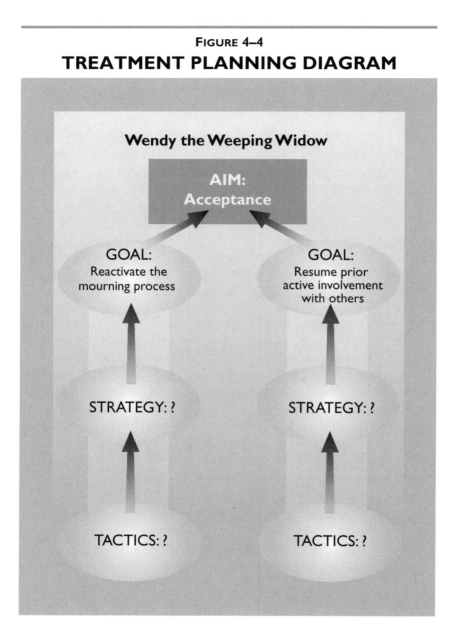

FIGURE 4–4

TREATMENT PLANNING DIAGRAM

EXAMPLE 5: PABLO THE PANICKED PAINTER

A 37-year-old bachelor, Pablo pursues married women for the sake of conquest and breaks off any relationship that threatens to become serious.[6] From a psychoanalytic point of view, the conquest of an idealized, apparently unattainable woman, becoming at least for the moment her choice over all rival men, suggests Pablo is acting out an oedipal fantasy. He projects characteristics on the women he courts that do not reflect who they really are; he sees them as idealized versions of his father's wife. In these substitute relationships, he gains his mother against his powerful rival, her husband. Our AIM here is loosely described as *achieve a mature love relationship.* Difficult to define, we might say it would be a committed and continuing relationship based on a realistic knowledge of the partner. For Pablo, we hope to replace this fantasy-based pattern with a more stable and realistic one. That partner might be Phyllis, his longtime friend, or someone new. We do not expect that our therapy will necessarily continue until Pablo marries the perfect mate—only that he alters his basis for selecting a woman to love. This formulation points the way toward treatment decisions.

Our work might fall into two phases. First, we would expect to help Pablo see his infatuation pattern for what it is—a desperate struggle with a phase of his life now long past—and thereby set up a counterforce to it. Second, we hope to see him make choices appropriate to the criteria listed above: committed, continuing, realistic. In terms of (psychoanalytic) psychosexual development, we look for him to begin making genital object choices. These two phases may well overlap. They can be listed (Figure 4–5) as GOALS: 1) eliminate inappropriate (oedipal) object choices and 2) achieve appropriate (genital) object choices.

DISCUSSION OF GOALS

Setting GOALS or objectives is a more familiar planning exercise than selecting the AIM or overall outcome of therapy. Even those who are strong advocates of treatment planning may consider the selection of GOALS the end of the planning process (Nurcombe 1987). A simple listing of GOALS, however, without the organizing principle provided by their

---

[6]See case vignette, Chapter 3, page 35.

FIGURE 4–5

TREATMENT PLANNING DIAGRAM

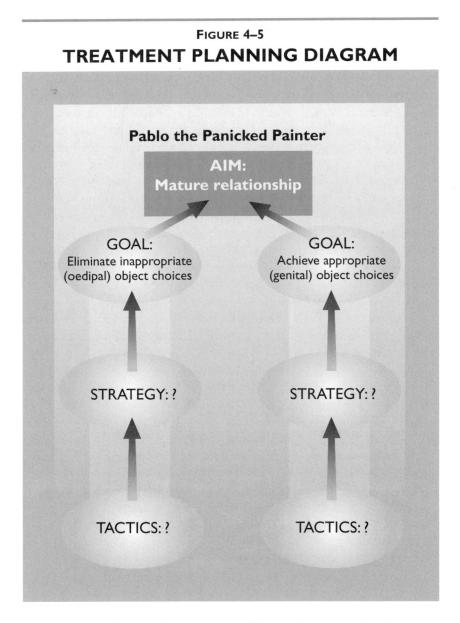

Pablo the Panicked Painter

AIM:
Mature relationship

GOAL:
Eliminate inappropriate
(oedipal) object choices

GOAL:
Achieve appropriate
(genital) object choices

STRATEGY: ?

STRATEGY: ?

TACTICS: ?

TACTICS: ?

relationship to the overall outcome, still leaves the plan unfinished.

Some GOALS on the list, even though they represent the patient's legitimate problems, may have a lower priority than others. Some may even be irrelevant to the patient at the current time, no matter how important they might have been in the past. Without the AIM as a framework within which to evaluate the patient's presenting problems, it may be difficult to organize the treatment plan. Once the treatment is under way, attention to less important GOALS may siphon off energy and time needed for the central issues of the case.

Problems, GOALS, and *objectives* are terms in common use. Their exact meaning often depends on the context or on a particular definition. In this context, I emphasize four characteristics:

1. The GOAL should be *specific*—that is, it should clearly outline a single issue.
2. It should be *measurable*—that is, it should be subject to a set of defined parameters or objective standards.
3. It should be *relevant*—that is, it should represent the solution to a significant current problem.
4. It should be *achievable*—that is, it should be within the conjoint capabilities of the patient and therapist.

Ticho (1972), discussing termination issues in psychoanalysis, made a useful distinction between "treatment goals" and "life goals." The former represent accomplishments within the analysis itself, whereas life goals are considered the ongoing work of the patient. Patients' success in achieving their life goals can be enhanced by a successful period of analytic work, but after patients reach their treatment goals, treatment ends. Life goals should not determine the length of treatment. This distinction may help us define the GOALS within the framework set by the AIM. GOALS are selected as components of the AIM. They are the parts that add up to the whole, the final outcome of the therapy. The patient may have other goals, important ones, which are not related to the optimum result of our anticipated work in the therapy. We can leave them for a later period of treatment, if there is one, or, as Ticho suggested, for patients to solve on their own.

REFERENCES

Erikson EH: Childhood and Society. New York, WW Norton, 1950

Hamilton M: A rating scale for depression. J Neurol Neurosurg Psychiatry 23:56–62, 1960

Nurcombe B: Diagnostic reasoning and treatment planning: II. Treatment. Aust N Z J Psychiatry 21:483–490, 1987

Ticho EA: Termination of psychoanalysis: treatment goals, life goals. Psychoanal Q 41:315–333, 1972

Chapter 5

STRATEGIES

DEFINITION

STRATEGIES are the therapeutic approaches that can help the patient move toward a GOAL. I chose the term STRATEGY to emphasize that a therapeutic approach is intended to solve particular problems. It has direction and purpose, and it can be evaluated on the results it produces. Each STRATEGY corresponds to a treatment modality, such as insight-oriented therapy, psychopharmacology, or cognitive-behavioral therapy. A STRATEGY may be concerned with a single therapeutic objective, or GOAL. Alternatively, one STRATEGY may serve to reach two or more GOALS.

As an example of the STRATEGY selection process, look again at the case of Ernest the Edgy Engineer.[1] We decided on a cognitive STRATEGY to deal with his damaged self-image and on sexual counseling—a behavioral STRATEGY—to improve his sexual function. However, we might have selected a cognitive approach for both GOALS. In that event, although we would use the same therapeutic modality, we would pursue each GOAL independently. On one occasion we might discuss Ernest's sexual problem with attention to such issues as performance anxiety, the meaning of his sexual relationship, possible unresolved marital issues, and so forth. At another time the session might focus on his damaged professional image, and we might explore the specific events that led him to magnify his modest mistake into a sense of complete failure, as well as the relationship of his perfectionism and overresponsibility to his difficulties. The distinction is made by the therapist, who must be clear that there are

---

[1]See case vignette, Chapter 2, pages 19–20.

two separate GOALS and that each deserves appropriate attention. The timing of that attention will most often depend on the patient: Ernest may bring up the sexual issue in one session and his professional anxiety in another. The therapist should recognize either topic as an agreed focus of therapeutic work and pursue it with the selected STRATEGY.

It is important not to confuse the process with the outcome. The STRATEGY is our method of working with the patient. The GOAL is the expected result of using that method.

The therapist may become caught up in the strategic process itself, rather than as a means to an end, because of comfort, familiarity, intellectual gratification, or more personal, countertransference issues. The tendency to confuse STRATEGIES with GOALS is more common among less-experienced therapists, but any of us can drift across the line, especially when process holds out some intriguing challenge. The risk is that the therapist's energies may be controlled by the STRATEGY rather than by the GOAL, by the process rather than by the result of using that process. When the therapist pursues the process for its own sake rather than to help the patient reach the necessary GOALS and achieve the desired AIM, therapy becomes diluted, diverted, or stalled. Efficient therapy requires keeping one's eye on the GOAL at all times.

When the distinction between STRATEGY and GOAL is not clear, a STRATEGY may be identified by asking: What is the purpose of this therapeutic effort? It may be further differentiated from a GOAL by asking: Can it accomplish what I expect? Process has purpose. It is methodology employed with intention to attain a particular end.

EXAMPLE 1: DEREK THE DEPRESSED DENTIST

Our GOALS for Derek are to eliminate depressive symptoms, to regain family and community involvement, and to minimize recurrence risk.[2] These three GOALS require different therapeutic approaches. For symptomatic relief, we can best help Derek by attacking the presumed biological substrate—oversimplified as the neurotransmitter deficit—with one or more appropriate medications. To help him regain family and community involvement, we must deal with his withdrawal and hopelessness. Here cognitive therapy might be the best approach. For our third

---

[2]See case vignette, Chapter 3, pages 26–27.

GOAL—minimizing the risk of recurrence—we can use antidepressant medication, but note that the STRATEGY is long-term follow-up assessment instead of medication. Of course, Derek's continuing to take the medication will reduce the chance of another depression or, if it occurs, will ensure that it will be more mild and manageable, but medication maintenance is a TACTIC by which our STRATEGY of long-term follow-up assessment can be carried out.

For Derek's plan, then, we can summarize how these STRATEGIES fit in with our chosen GOALS (Table 5–1).

TABLE 5–1. Derek: goals and strategies

Goal	Strategy
Eliminate depressive symptoms	Psychopharmacology
Regain family and community involvement	Cognitive therapy
Minimize recurrence risk	Long-term follow-up assessment

Now we can replace the question marks in our planning diagram with these strategic decisions (Figure 5–1).

EXAMPLE 2: DOROTHY THE DESPAIRING DOWAGER

For Dorothy, an older woman struggling with the despair of what she perceives as an unfulfilled and meaningless life, the treatment GOALS are to confirm her nurturing role and to engage in meaningful work.[3] The STRATEGY that might be appropriate for both these GOALS is a transactional approach. A transactional therapist looks for a patient's life script, the apparent blueprint the patient has drawn up, without fully realizing it, to guide choices and outlook. The emphasis placed on her life choices and patterns might fit in quite well with Dorothy's need to reexamine her own life path and to help her see it still has purpose. We can add this STRATEGY to her treatment plan. As Figure 5–2 shows, we have replaced the outlined two-STRATEGY portion of the template with the single one we selected, and consequently, we now anticipate only a single set of TACTICS.

---

[3]See case vignette, Chapter 3, page 29.

FIGURE 5–1
TREATMENT PLANNING DIAGRAM

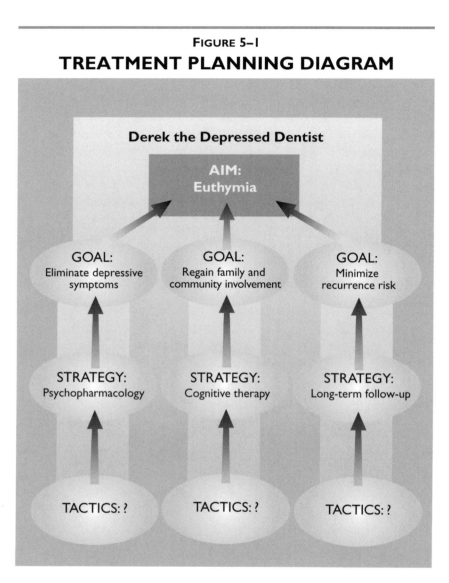

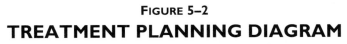

FIGURE 5–2

TREATMENT PLANNING DIAGRAM

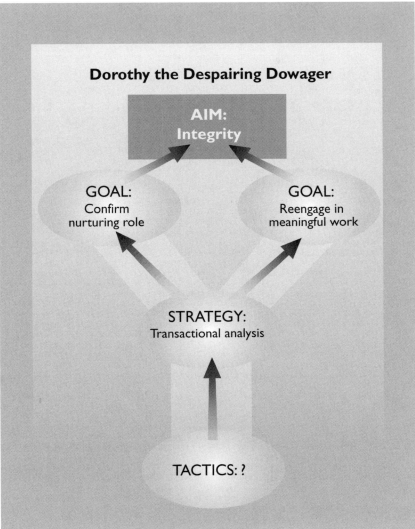

Dorothy the Despairing Dowager

AIM:
Integrity

GOAL:
Confirm
nurturing role

GOAL:
Reengage in
meaningful work

STRATEGY:
Transactional analysis

TACTICS: ?

EXAMPLE 3: ULYSSES THE UNEMPLOYED UNDERTAKER

We had three GOALS to help Ulysses resolve his situational crisis (the AIM) by reentering the workforce: symptom relief, social reengagement, and effective job seeking.[4] A psychopharmacological STRATEGY could prove helpful with two of them. Symptomatic relief might be achieved with a prescribed medication designed to replace his use of alcohol. (The premise that he is self-medicating with alcohol is based on our formulation, an element of the planning process whose importance cannot be overemphasized.) It may be that one medication may benefit Ulysses with regard to our second GOAL, social reengagement. We will look at the question of which particular medication to use in our consideration of TACTICS, but for the sake of clarity let me mention it here as well. An anxiety-reducing (anxiolytic) medication not only might substitute for the alcohol but also might reverse his increased avoidance of social situations. Here, one STRATEGY would be employed in reaching two GOALS.

With regard to the social anxiety, however, medication alone would likely not be sufficient. A second STRATEGY to help him reduce his social avoidance might incorporate a behavioral approach. One reason for this choice is our assessment that Ulysses is not very psychologically minded, but he is motivated to change, and he may be responsive to direct suggestions about how to attack these problems.

Our third GOAL, effective job seeking, could be pursued through a case management approach. We could serve as a resource of information on where and how to get help with finding a new job.

Figure 5–3 places these STRATEGIES in our planning diagram.

EXAMPLE 4: WENDY THE WEEPING WIDOW

The GOALS we thought might help Wendy accept her husband's death were to facilitate the mourning process and to resume her prior active involvement with others.[5] Her withdrawal, isolation, and prolonged bereavement have kept her life on hold for 3 years. If the therapist takes an active role, it might be difficult to confront her with the issues she is try-

---

[4]See case vignette, Chapter 3, page 31.

[5]See case vignette, Chapter 3, page 33.

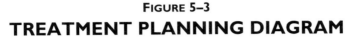

FIGURE 5–3
TREATMENT PLANNING DIAGRAM

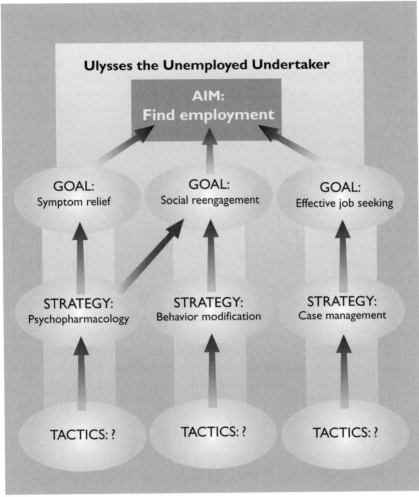

ing to avoid. Therapists have different personal styles, and some might welcome the challenge of breaking into Wendy's pathological way of coping with her loss. In my judgment, the risk that she would become so distressed she would leave therapy would outweigh the chances of success with a confrontational approach.

An alternative approach would use the type of therapy developed by Rogers (1951), an approach that falls within the general category of existential therapy. Early on, Rogers called his system "nondirective therapy," but in later writings he amended the name to "client-centered therapy" and finally to "person-centered therapy." The core concept of existential therapy, which contains ideas some would call philosophical or even religious, is that the therapist should "be with" the patient. By accepting what patients say at face value (instead of looking for underlying meaning) and by using empathic listening to try to feel what patients feel, the therapist expects that patients will find their own way toward healing. Rogers's approach builds on these techniques, and I refer to them more specifically in the discussion of TACTICS. Suffice it here to say that a Rogerian approach seems to offer a less distressing kind of therapy experience for this vulnerable woman and would be a reasonable choice of STRATEGY.

I would anticipate that the nondirective approach would be sufficient to help Wendy with our first GOAL of facilitating the mourning process. I think it will also contribute helpfully to the second, because she could be expected to resume some of her prior relationships as she worked her way through her grief. I am not sure she would wholly succeed with the nondirective work alone, and I would therefore add a second STRATEGY, most likely timing its use later in the course of the therapy, to help her more actively with the GOAL of getting reinvolved in social relationships. This second STRATEGY—let us simply call it a directive approach—might seem contradictory to my argument for a nonconfrontational therapy. Clearly, one cannot act both ways at once, and whatever directive measures are employed must provoke as little anxiety as possible. It would require judgment to know when to use the more directive STRATEGY and just how directive it would be wise to be. That being said, sometimes there is no better intervention than some plain-spoken advice.

The larger point is that you can use different STRATEGIES—even those that seem incompatible—over the course of therapy. If you select the best STRATEGY to reach the GOALS you have set, if you have the requisite skills and experience with each therapeutic modality you intend to use, and if you time the use of each STRATEGY judiciously, the patient will benefit from the wider selection that you offer.

For Wendy, then, we plan on using the two STRATEGIES reflected in Figure 5–4.

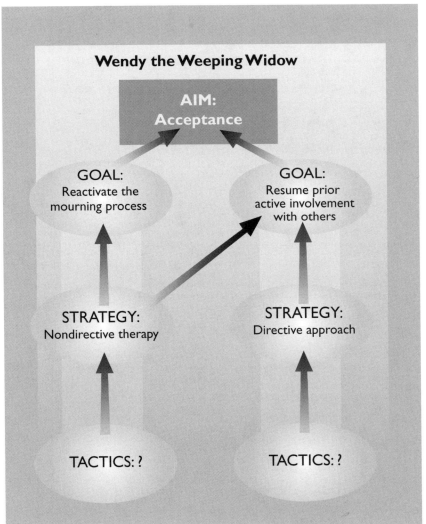

FIGURE 5–4

TREATMENT PLANNING DIAGRAM

Wendy the Weeping Widow

**AIM:
Acceptance**

GOAL:
Reactivate the
mourning process

GOAL:
Resume prior
active involvement
with others

STRATEGY:
Nondirective therapy

STRATEGY:
Directive approach

TACTICS: ?

TACTICS: ?

EXAMPLE 5: PABLO THE PANICKED PAINTER

Our previous planning effort for Pablo yielded two related GOALS that together, if achieved, could help this anxious artist find his way to at least one mature relationship: to eliminate inappropriate (oedipal) object choices and to achieve appropriate (genital) object choices.[6] Given the psychodynamic formulation we used to define these GOALS, our therapeutic modality ought to be psychodynamic psychotherapy.

Perhaps it is worth making the distinctions again between a GOAL and a STRATEGY and between STRATEGY and TACTICS, using this case as an illustration. Suppose we took the second GOAL and worded it: "support and assist appropriate (genital) object choices"? Would we still have defined a GOAL? We would not. Our original statement used the word *achieve* to define the GOAL. To achieve the desired result is to reach an end point, to complete an objective. When we say instead "support and assist" the appropriate choice of a partner, we are describing elements of the process by which we intend to help Pablo get to the desired GOAL. The distinction between end point and process helps us distinguish GOAL from STRATEGY. Then, if "support and assist" does not define a GOAL, does it constitute a STRATEGY? No again. Supportive measures are techniques. Winston et al. (1986) reviewed the history and relevance of this diverse concept. They concluded, "Most authors agree that supportive psychotherapy is not so much a modality of therapy as it is a body of techniques and attitudes that are present to a greater or lesser extent in any psychotherapeutic endeavor" (p. 1113). We might use supportive measures to some degree with Pablo's therapy, even with our intended expressive, insight-oriented approach. If we adopted one of the more directive therapies, our support and assistance would likely play a much larger part in our work with him. For example, we might support Pablo's choice of an appropriate love interest, if he were to make such a choice, by giving helpful advice or praising his actions. Regardless of whether the supportive measures are minimal or constitute the bulk of the work, they remain technical elements in the therapy. In the planning process, they would be regarded as TACTICS.

To summarize: A GOAL is an end point. A STRATEGY is a process. A TACTIC is a technique.

Now let us place the selected STRATEGY on our planning diagram for Pablo (Figure 5–5).

---

[6]See case vignette, Chapter 3, page 35.

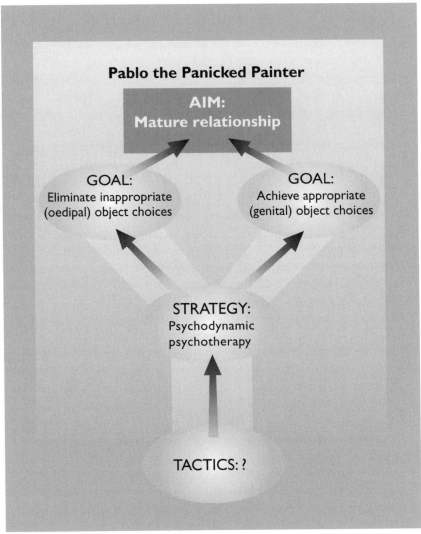

FIGURE 5–5
TREATMENT PLANNING DIAGRAM

Pablo the Panicked Painter

AIM:
Mature relationship

GOAL:
Eliminate inappropriate
(oedipal) object choices

GOAL:
Achieve appropriate
(genital) object choices

STRATEGY:
Psychodynamic
psychotherapy

TACTICS: ?

DISCUSSION OF STRATEGIES

In presenting a number of treatment plans, I have used different types of psychotherapy within a single plan and suggested a wider variety among the several examples. The use of multiple treatment modalities is a complex issue. On the level of theory, as expressed in the literature and in educational programs, tension exists between the idea that one or another school of psychotherapy is sufficient to handle most or all treatment and the contrary idea that some combination or amalgam of psychotherapies is necessary. On the level of practice, clinicians may restrict themselves to the techniques of a single psychotherapy, or they may achieve competence in several.

Since the early twentieth century, physicists have pursued a mathematical quest for the "unified theory" that would bring all natural forces, including gravity, together within a single, coherent formula. Less ambitious efforts in psychotherapy research have tried to unify two or more treatments, crossing the spectrum from biological through psychodynamic to social and existential, into a single, coherent whole. *Eclecticism* (Simon 1974), *differential therapeutics* (Frances et al. 1984), and *integrative psychotherapy* (Beitman et al. 1989) all refer to some of these efforts. Some of the more successful efforts include cognitive-analytic therapy, dialectical-behavior therapy, and psychodynamic-interpersonal therapy. (Holmes and Bateman 2002) In the practical realm of day-to-day clinical work, therapists often cross the boundaries of theory to select and use what they feel is most effective and best for the patient. This selective use has been called technical eclecticism (Lazarus 1967).

The use of multiple therapies may take one of at least three forms:

1. The therapist might bring together his or her own combination of selected techniques from different types of therapies. One example might be the theoretical approach of psychodynamic therapy, a communicative style combining Rogerian and cognitive elements, and interventions that are a mixture of supportive and interpretative statements. Another example is the therapist with a behavioral orientation who begins with a concrete set of behavioral interventions—relaxation exercises and in vivo desensitization, for example—but who gradually shifts to a psychodynamic frame of reference and begins to focus on aspects of the patient's relationship with and attitude toward the therapist. These examples show the blending process through which a therapist might develop a personal style that can be adapted to a wide variety of clinical challenges (Havens 1973).

2. A second type of multiple-treatment approach requires the therapist to have a working knowledge of a spectrum of separate therapies (Abroms 1983). Here the therapist has several therapeutic options but chooses the one that seems best suited to a particular patient's needs and sticks to it throughout a single course of therapy. The therapist might elect to work with one patient in the framework of trans-

actional analysis, take a cognitive approach with another, and use group therapy with a third. The therapist might instead begin with one therapy (perhaps directive, to resolve a presenting crisis), and then switch to another (family therapy, for instance) after the first has been successful. Any of the available psychotherapies might include the use of medication as indicated by the patient's condition. Except for combining it with psychopharmacology, the therapist tries to remain consistent with a single type of therapy throughout a period of work with the patient.

3. A third approach may use different therapeutic modalities in treating a single patient. Two or more therapeutic approaches are used at the same time, with the therapist switching from one to the other as the flow of treatment requires. This multimodal approach (Lazarus 1981) would seem to place the greatest demands on the therapist, but the ability to select among a number of distinct therapeutic modalities affords the therapist greater range and flexibility and promises better results with a greater variety of patients and a wider array of clinical challenges.

REFERENCES

Abroms EM: Beyond eclecticism. Am J Psychiatry 140:740–745, 1983

Beitman BD, Goldfried MR, Norcross JC: The movement toward integrating the psychotherapies: an overview. Am J Psychiatry 146:138–147, 1989

Frances A, Clarkin J, Perry S: Differential Therapeutics in Psychiatry: The Art and Science of Treatment Selection. New York, Brunner/Mazel, 1984

Havens LL: Approaches to the Mind: Movement of the Psychiatric Schools From Sects Toward Science. Boston, MA, Little, Brown, 1973

Holmes J, Bateman AW: Integration in Psychotherapy: Models and Methods. New York, Oxford University Press, 2002

Lazarus AA: In support of technical eclecticism. Psychol Rep 21:415–416, 1967

Lazarus AA: The Practice of Multimodal Therapy: Systematic, Comprehensive, and Effective Psychotherapy. New York, McGraw-Hill, 1981

Rogers CR: Client-Centered Therapy: Its Current Practice, Implications and Theory. Boston, MA, Houghton Mifflin, 1951

Simon RM: On eclecticism. Am J Psychiatry 131:135–139, 1974

Winston A, Pinsker H, McCullough L: A review of supportive psychotherapy. Hosp Community Psychiatry 37:1107–1114, 1986

Chapter 6

TACTICS

DEFINITION

TACTICS are the therapeutic interventions that implement a STRATEGY, the techniques by which the therapist helps the patient move forward in the strategic effort to reach a necessary goal. They attempt to influence the patient's behavior directly—for example, by the behavioral prescription of desensitization exercises—or indirectly—for example, by offering insightful interpretations. A TACTIC is usually employed more than once.

Just as all STRATEGIES are not psychotherapeutic modalities, so not all TACTICS involve psychotherapy techniques. Psychopharmacology is a STRATEGY whose TACTICS would include anxiolytics, neuroleptics, antidepressants, and other psychoactive medications. Case management is another example of a nontherapy STRATEGY. Its implementation would include such TACTICS as use of community resources, supervision of supportive living arrangements, and vocational help.

To discuss the technical interventions employed in the multitude of psychotherapies is well beyond the scope of this book. Each of the many psychotherapies has a number of variations and progeny, and each of those has its own technical requirements. Although I have had to reduce complex technical efforts to a deceptively simple list of terms, I assume the reader is familiar with these techniques or has access to sources describing them.

EXAMPLE 1: DEREK THE DEPRESSED DENTIST

Our STRATEGY to eliminate Derek's depressive symptoms[1] is psychopharmacology, and the TACTIC would be, naturally, an antidepressant

---

[1]See case vignette, Chapter 3, pages 26–27.

FIGURE 6–1

TREATMENT PLANNING DIAGRAM

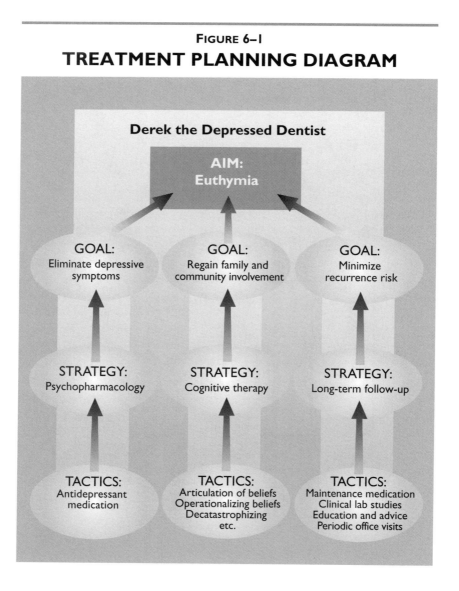

Derek the Depressed Dentist

AIM: Euthymia

GOAL:	GOAL:	GOAL:
Eliminate depressive symptoms	Regain family and community involvement	Minimize recurrence risk

STRATEGY:	STRATEGY:	STRATEGY:
Psychopharmacology	Cognitive therapy	Long-term follow-up

TACTICS:	TACTICS:	TACTICS:
Antidepressant medication	Articulation of beliefs Operationalizing beliefs Decatastrophizing etc.	Maintenance medication Clinical lab studies Education and advice Periodic office visits

medication. Tactical choices would also include which antidepressant to use, its dosage, possible augmentation of the primary medication with a second agent, how to monitor compliance, and other considerations.

We selected cognitive therapy to help Derek overcome his withdrawal from family, friends, and community activities. Its approach contrasts the patient's logical inconsistencies and misperceptions with realistic and factual alternatives and thereby attempts to weaken and eliminate the symptoms they support. Cognitive TACTICS we might consider in working with Derek would include "articulation of beliefs, operationalizing beliefs, decentering, decatastrophizing, challenging the 'shoulds,' challenging beliefs through behavioral exercises, perspective hypothesis testing, and reattribution techniques" (Garner 1989, p. 542).

Our final STRATEGY is long-term follow-up assessment to minimize the risk of recurrent depression. The key tactical intervention would be to have Derek continue taking the antidepressant medication after his acute condition had cleared. As another TACTIC, we might try to enhance his compliance by advising him of the risk of recurrence and educating him about the research that supports this recommendation. We can now complete our planning diagram for Derek (Figure 6–1).

EXAMPLE 2: DOROTHY THE DESPAIRING DOWAGER

We decided on a single STRATEGY—transactional analysis—to try to help Dorothy achieve a sense of integrity about her life situation through nurturing others and through resuming some type of meaningful work.[2] The premise of transactional analysis (Berne 1961) is that three *ego states* may influence a person's feelings, ideas, and behavior: the Parent, the Adult, and the Child. Functional problems arise when the Adult is contaminated by one of the other two or when one of the three states is excluded. The therapist tries to identify *games*, in which these dysfunctional transactions are played out between the patient and other people, and *scripts*, or lifelong patterns of dysfunctional interactions. Interventions try to help the patient strengthen the Adult. One way to do this is by exposing *crossed transactions*, in which, for instance, tension arises between the Adult state of one person and the Parental state of another.

Putting these TACTICS into our treatment diagram completes our plan for Dorothy (Figure 6–2).

---

[2]See case vignette, Chapter 3, page 29.

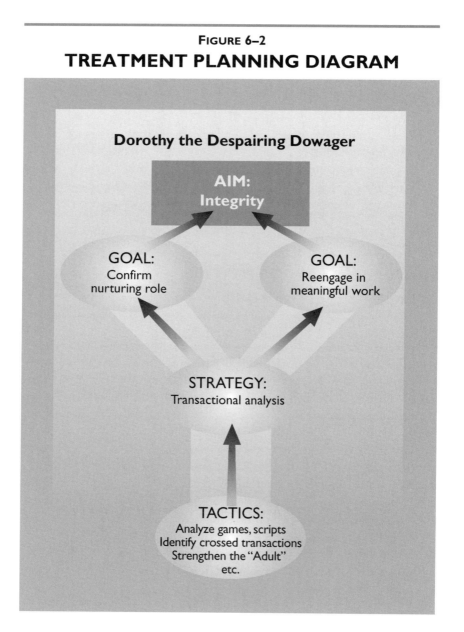

FIGURE 6–2

TREATMENT PLANNING DIAGRAM

EXAMPLE 3: ULYSSES THE UNEMPLOYED UNDERTAKER

We selected three different STRATEGIES to pursue the three GOALS we think will help Ulysses reach the relatively modest AIM of returning to work.[3] We expected one of the STRATEGIES, psychopharmacology, to be helpful both in providing symptom relief (GOAL 1) and in reducing his social anxiety (part of GOAL 2). The tactical considerations include selection of medication, dosage, side effects, interactions with other concurrent medicines, risk–benefit ratio, and all the other factors that determine the selection of the best medication for a particular patient. A reasonable choice would be a single (nonaddicting) anxiolytic agent, perhaps a selective serotonin reuptake inhibitor, both to reduce his general anxiety so that he would not need alcohol for this purpose and to blunt the specific anxiety he is experiencing in social situations.

A second STRATEGY, behavior modification, might help him overcome his social anxiety. Technique in behavior therapy includes learning new, specific ways of dealing with internal and external stresses that can replace the ineffective, symptom-producing habits the patient brings to therapy. Behavioral techniques might include relaxation training (Wolpe 1979), imagery techniques (Cautela 1979), modeling (Bandura 1969), desensitization (Wolpe 1958), and assertiveness training (Wolpe 1979).

Our third STRATEGY was case management. The tactical means to carry out this approach may be somewhat restricted for office-based practitioners, but they might include discussing his vocational interests and plans, suggesting use of the help-wanted section of the newspaper, and other simple measures. We could also consider referring Ulysses to an outside agency for vocational counseling, testing, and placement. The referral itself would be a tactical decision, but we would need to weigh the possible benefit against the chance his social anxiety and even his drinking might make it difficult for him to cooperate with such a program. We would remain involved with the outside agencies, perhaps serving in a liaison capacity.

These tactical choices allow us to complete the planning diagram for Ulysses' initial treatment (Figure 6–3).

---

[3]See case vignette, Chapter 3, page 31.

FIGURE 6–3
TREATMENT PLANNING DIAGRAM

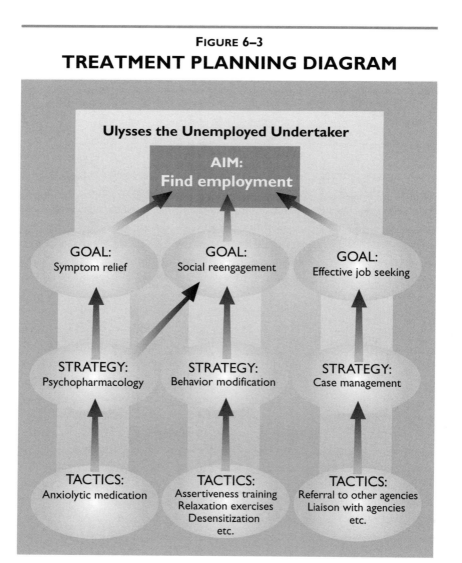

Ulysses the Unemployed Undertaker

AIM:
Find employment

GOAL: Symptom relief

GOAL: Social reengagement

GOAL: Effective job seeking

STRATEGY: Psychopharmacology

STRATEGY: Behavior modification

STRATEGY: Case management

TACTICS: Anxiolytic medication

TACTICS: Assertiveness training
Relaxation exercises
Desensitization
etc.

TACTICS: Referral to other agencies
Liaison with agencies
etc.

EXAMPLE 4: WENDY THE WEEPING WIDOW

Sometimes TACTICS, as a set of teachable techniques, are hard to define. A prime example of this difficulty is existential psychotherapy. Havens (1974) offered a definition on "the existential use of the self." He described the core of the existential method as the effort of the therapist to be where the patient is—in other words, to remove the boundary between them as much as possible. He recommended techniques such as "keeping looking," taking everything the patient says at face value, and avoiding the natural inclination to come to a conclusion about what motivates the patient. These TACTICS allow the therapist to stay with the other person's immediate conscious state and to encourage the patient's innate healing power.

The STRATEGY for Wendy[4] anticipated we would use the approach developed by Rogers (1951). Technically, the patient is allowed to do most of the talking. The therapist sometimes restates what the patient has said to reflect the feelings and ideas the patient may not yet fully appreciate. Other TACTICS involve an unquestioning acceptance of the patient, "unconditional positive regard," empathic understanding, and congruence with the patient's position and outlook, all part of the effort to "stay with the patient."

We anticipated a more active STRATEGY, a more directive approach that might be useful later in the therapy. The TACTICS involved would simply be the judicious use of advice and suggestion.

Completing our treatment planning for Wendy now gives us the diagram in Figure 6–4.

---

[4]See case vignette, Chapter 3, page 33.

FIGURE 6–4

TREATMENT PLANNING DIAGRAM

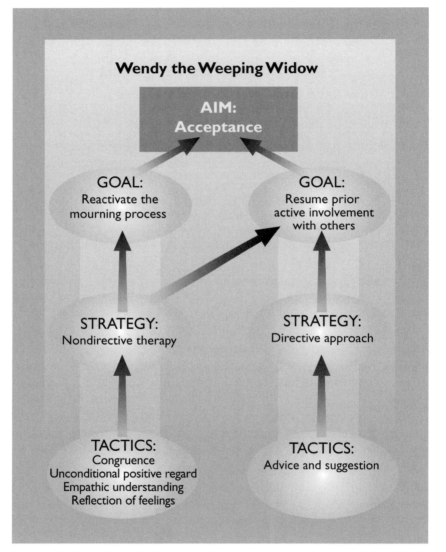

EXAMPLE 5: PABLO THE PANICKED PAINTER

Our STRATEGY to help Pablo become capable of mature relationships through substituting at least one appropriate choice of partner for his current string of inappropriate partners was psychodynamic psychotherapy.[5] Freud's main TACTIC, early in his development of psychoanalysis, was "making the unconscious conscious." Some of his early analyses were quite short, perhaps a few weeks on the couch while Freud gathered the data from which he could deduce the unconscious meaning of the symptom. His expectation was that simply telling this to the patient would make the patient better. Indeed, it seemed to work at first. Later Freud acknowledged patients must come on the insight themselves, a process that took considerably longer (Hendricks 1966).

The tactical sequence in classical psychoanalysis might be captured aphoristically in three stages: remembering, repeating, and working through. The patient *remembers* through freely associating on the couch. The patient *repeats* through the development of the transference neurosis: the repetition, with the analyst as object, of perceptions and feelings originally generated within familial and other early close relationships. *Working through* results from repeated exposure to these remembered and recreated experiences, from the interpretations of the analyst and from the resulting production of new material by the analysand. Although psychodynamic psychotherapy may have the same strategic focus—to help the patient develop insight that will catalyze helpful change—it relies less on the transference neurosis and allows the therapist a less neutral role.

Tactically, the work often proceeds in a four- or five-step sequence: 1) identification, 2) clarification, 3) confrontation, 4) interpretation, and 5) working through.

Initially, the therapist tries to identify a problem area. Once the area has been detected, the next effort is to clarify it through direct inquiry and active listening. The therapist may offer an interpretation. There follows a period of further working through the interpretative idea to achieve its full effect and potential. Between the clarification of an issue and the offer of interpretation, the therapist may sometimes confront the patient with the problem.

In the case of our panicked painter, we would want to establish, through the history and active listening, the psychodynamic basis for his

---

[5]See case vignette, Chapter 3, page 35.

FIGURE 6–5

TREATMENT PLANNING DIAGRAM

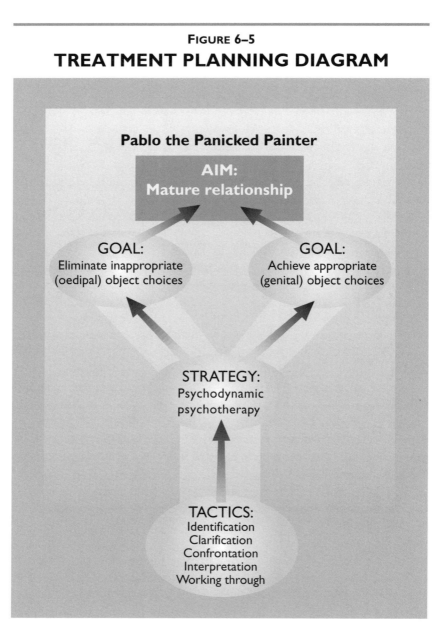

Pablo the Panicked Painter

AIM:
Mature relationship

GOAL:
Eliminate inappropriate
(oedipal) object choices

GOAL:
Achieve appropriate
(genital) object choices

STRATEGY:
Psychodynamic
psychotherapy

TACTICS:
Identification
Clarification
Confrontation
Interpretation
Working through

promiscuous behavior. Greatly oversimplified, this process would begin with our formulation that suggests we will listen for evidence to support the self-defeating nature of Pablo's pursuit of married women (identification). We may have to point out to Pablo, using his own description of their frustrating course, just how self-defeating these relationships are for him (confrontation). We will follow up any such leads with active exploration of these issues (clarification). When we think we hear parallels between these triangular relationships and what he might have told us about his childhood frustrations with his parents, we may try to connect them (interpretation). As we continue to listen, we expect further material to emerge and be experienced, interpreted, and discussed (working through). The insight he gains, it is hoped, will allow Pablo to inhibit his inclination to seek triangular relationships and instead to cast his eye on a woman more suitable for a mature relationship—that is, a relationship without the emotional baggage of childhood wishes that can never be realized. When he does, our same STRATEGY and its TACTICS should be able to support his fledgling efforts to seek these new relationships.

Putting all of this into our treatment diagram, we now see the final plan for Pablo (Figure 6–5).

DISCUSSION OF TACTICS

Although they occupy most of the time and energy of a therapy already in progress, tactical considerations are the least important element of the planning process. In our top-down approach, designating the AIM is most important. Deriving from that AIM the GOALS that will make it happen is the second step, one that requires careful analysis and creative thinking. Strategic choices depend on the therapist's training and experience to provide a solid working knowledge of which therapeutic modalities can best achieve the proposed result. TACTICS follow almost automatically from the designation of a STRATEGY.

TACTICS are the stuff of clinical anecdote, the focus of curbstone consultation, the warp and woof of supervision, and they seem to engage a large portion of the energy and attention involved in the decision of what to do with the patient. They are often the focus of case conferences in which a therapist presents a problematic case and one or more colleagues offer suggestions, all of which use some TACTIC, a specific approach or maneuver. Each commentator may have his or her own GOALS in mind or even have a notion about the desired outcome, but the failure to enunciate these more inclusive therapeutic levels can seriously undermine the effort to help. Instead, the entire conference can become mired in a confusing welter of contradictory or dead-end suggestions. This emphasis on TACTICS is often misplaced and may even distort the conduct of psychotherapy. If Napoleon had planned his campaigns by paying attention only to horsemanship, close-order drill, and the use of the bayonet, he would have been defeated long before Waterloo. Like all great generals, Napoleon chose the objective (the AIM) of his campaign, then engaged the enemy in the battles (GOALS) that would bring that objective to fruition. When he saw the lay of the land and the strength of the opposing forces, he designed a STRATEGY to win the battle, and only then did he decide on the troop deployments, armor, and munitions (TACTICS) needed to carry the day.

In psychotherapy planning, once settled on a STRATEGY, the choice of TACTICS follows, based on training and experience. Judgment and timing will determine how and when to employ each therapeutic element. Therapists may choose to construct a genogram, suggest assigned exercises between sessions, accompany the patient into a phobia-inducing environment, interpret a recent dream, question an interpersonal game, or challenge a negative overgeneralization, as long as the intervention is appropriate to the therapeutic framework.

Just as the potential to select among diverse STRATEGIES favors the therapist who is comfortable with a variety of therapeutic approaches and the techniques of each, the choice of TACTICS for a particular therapy with a particular patient depends on a broad grounding in the wide field of psychotherapy. Diversity and flexibility are the hallmarks of the ability to deal successfully with a wide spectrum of patients presenting with a variety of problems.

REFERENCES

Bandura A: Principles of Behavior Modification. New York, Holt, Rinehart and Winston, 1969

Berne E: Transactional Analysis in Psychotherapy: A Systematic Individual and Social Psychiatry. New York, Grove, 1961

Cautela JR: Covert Conditioning. New York, Pergamon, 1979

Garner D: Cognitive therapy, in Treatments of Psychiatric Disorders: A Task Force Report of the American Psychiatric Association, Vol 1. Washington, DC, American Psychiatric Association, 1989, pp 537–542

Havens LL: The existential use of the self. Am J Psychiatry 131:1–10, 1974

Hendricks I: Facts and Theories of Psychoanalysis, 3rd Edition. New York, Dell, 1966

Rogers CR: Client-Centered Therapy: Its Current Practice, Implications and Theory. Boston, MA, Houghton Mifflin, 1951

Wolpe J: Psychotherapy by Reciprocal Inhibition. Stanford, CA, Stanford University Press, 1958

Wolpe J: The Practice of Behavior Therapy, 3rd Edition. New York, Pergamon, 1979

Chapter 7

FORMULATION

The Critical Step in Treatment Planning

The formulation is the linchpin of treatment planning. More than a summary of the case, it is a synthesis of the patient's history, current problems, and signs and symptoms into a set of ideas from which treatment decisions can emerge.

At its simplest level, a formulation is an explanation of why the patient has the problems that brought him or her to the therapist. It describes the key features of the history and tries to link them in a meaningful way by discerning cause-and-effect relationships between past and present, between conflicts and symptoms. If successful, it organizes the clinical picture and allows the therapist to make predictions about future behavior and the course of treatment. Ultimately, the formulation is the basis for deriving the AIM and the GOALS that are the essence of treatment planning.

Yet most clinicians seem reluctant to use this part of the evaluation process and either do not formulate their cases at all or simply begin the initial therapy with a few ideas obtained from the initial assessment. Their formulations are rarely made a formal part of the patient's record. Perry et al. (1987), arguing that all of the reasons for this reluctance are unfounded, posited five misconceptions that underlay the omissions. They suggested that clinicians believe formulations are only useful in long-term therapy; that they want to avoid an elaborate and time-consuming process; that they view the process as merely a training exercise, one an experienced therapist no longer needs; that they view a formulation as something that could be constructed just as well "in one's head" as written into the patient's record; or that they believe that if they invest energy in a formulation, they will not pay attention to patient communications that do not fit their formulation.

Less experienced psychotherapists, lacking a clear concept of formulation, may form a diagnostic impression without a general sense of the therapy task before them and may believe they have formulated the case when in fact they have only given a summary description of it. More experienced therapists may have a different problem, treating the formulation as a good-enough element of their work. If at the end of the assessment they have some ideas about why the patient is behaving problematically, they may go no further and instead may push on into treatment before they have fully exploited these conclusions and considered the treatment objectives they should generate. Closing off the effort prematurely in that manner can point the therapy at issues of lesser importance, and once the therapy goes astray or meanders down a side path leading to a dead end, it is very difficult to get it back on track.

The central importance of formulation has been widely recognized. Some have advocated a highly structured, almost formulaic approach (Eells 1997) that is perhaps more useful for regulatory and third-party payment issues than as a basis for treatment planning. Others have illustrated the differences in formulating a case within different "psychiatric orientations," such as psychodynamic, biological, behavioral, and biopsychosocial perspectives (Sperry et al. 1992). How therapists construct the formulation varies with their theoretical preferences. The psychodynamic therapist will think about deficits or early conflicts and how they generated symptoms. The behaviorist will look at antecedent forces and their consequences and will pay attention to the contingencies that maintain symptomatic behavior. The transactionalist will consider the patient's interactions with other individuals and with groups of significant others. Those comfortable with other theoretical constructs will show similar diversity in formulating the case. Horowitz (1997) offered an integrative approach, using psychodynamic, interpersonal, cognitive-behavioral, and family systems concepts, organized around states of mind, patterns of conscious experience, and interpersonal expression, to address the question "What can this patient change now?"

The old story applies here of the blind men describing the elephant differently depending on which part of it they touch, but the language and the concepts used to construct the formulation are less important than the use made of the result. Whatever the theoretical framework, the ideas about the patient are likely to be congruent even if the terminology differs. The utility of the formulation will depend more on the creative energy of the therapist than on the form in which it is expressed.

A formulation begins with a short descriptive summary of the case, including the formal diagnosis. After that should come a series of hypotheses to explain what is wrong with the patient, how he or she got that way, and what might be the key areas on which therapy could focus. The idea is to highlight and clarify the central issues and to minimize those not immediately important.

In my experience, the single most common failing in formulating a case is to summarize it and stop. The summary is merely a listing of the clinical facts with no attempt to order them in a way that suggests what course of action might be helpful. A summary will not suffice. For example, one might describe Derek, the dentist we discussed earlier,[1] as depressed and unable to function within his family and community. One might add that his sleep, appetite, energy, and concentration are all diminished, and he has thoughts of suicide. This brief list reveals little to guide the therapy. If the formulation is to provide a basis for treatment planning, it must offer an explanation, based on cause-and-effect reasoning, of how and why the patient developed the problems therapy is to address. The formulation must also provide answers as to why the patient came to *us*, why now, and what the patient wants from therapy.

The case of Pablo, the painter with a penchant for married women,[2] can serve as an example. A descriptive summary would only report that Pablo pursues a seemingly unending series of women but loses interest once his pursuit succeeds, leaving him, at age 37, dissatisfied, a man whose emotional life seems stalled and ultimately empty. The formulation we began in our discussion of GOAL selection went further. We attempted to explain Pablo's behavior as a repetitive quest for a woman like his mother. We suggested that each of his conquests is an effort to displace his father and that his relationships fail when the reality of the women he seduces clashes too strongly with the romanticized ideal he is seeking. In short, Pablo is acting out a fantasy—for simplicity we can call it an oedipal fantasy—no longer relevant to a man in his 30s. This explanation may be only partially correct or it may be wrong; at this early stage of our work with him, we have only a limited amount of information, but even these preliminary conclusions can generate an effective treatment plan.

Any formulation is subject to revision as more data become available. That next revision might be revised again as still more of the story

---

[1] See case vignette, Chapter 3, pages 26–27.
[2] See case vignette, Chapter 3, page 35.

unfolds. A formulation is merely a snapshot of a particular moment in time, an attempt to represent what we know up to that moment in the most accurate and encompassing way we can, and our subsequent efforts will also strive to be as accurate and complete as possible. In this way, the formulation process creates a *dynamic model* of the patient, evolving over time.

History teaches us that scientific models need constant expansion, correction, or revision and may sometimes be discarded altogether, as new findings emerge. Ptolemy and his predecessors held that the Earth was the center of the universe and that the sun and planets revolved around it. When Copernicus proposed that the planets circle the sun, his revision required new observations—additional data—for final proof. Later observations placed our solar system within a galaxy, and current theory suggests that all heavenly bodies are being propelled outward from the center of a primordial explosion. No doubt the Big Bang theory will be further revised, perhaps even radically changed, as new data accrue from later scientific observation.

Medical history provides a similar illustration. Early explanations of disease relied on the suspected influences of angered gods and evil spirits. The ancient Greeks advanced to a theory that health and illness resulted from the balance among four humors: blood, phlegm, yellow bile, and black bile. As the Christian era began, Galen added anatomic knowledge to the humoral theory and brought scientific method to the art of medicine. Centuries later, Paracelsus quashed the humoral theory and inaugurated the modern medical era. New observations were the source of these and every subsequent advance of medical progress. New data revise medical models. A formulation, like a scientific model, represents the best explanation available at the time. Like medical models, a series of formulations will be successive approximations of the truth.

THE ROLE OF INDUCTIVE LOGIC

Successful recognition of the AIM and of the GOALS in a treatment plan depends heavily on the ability of the planner to use an inductive reasoning process. Inductive logic requires us to abstract from a group of apparently unrelated facts the idea that unifies them into a single concept. For example, confronted with an apple, a pear, and an orange, we can find a unifying concept by recognizing that all three are fruit. If we add a fourth item, a tomato, the concept *fruit* still applies, but we must know that a tomato is a fruit, not a vegetable. Adding a fifth item, a carrot, which is a vegetable, requires a new concept: say, *edible plants*. Another addition—a chicken—enlarges the concept further; the group now contains both plant and animal members. Perhaps *food* would cover them all. As more items with different characteristics enter the group, the overall inclusive concept becomes more difficult to recognize. Add to the above six items a sponge mop and a package of garbage bags; the category might be *supermarket items*. If instead we add a cat, a frog, and an earthworm, the category now could be *living things*.

In clinical assessment, we acquire a large number of items of information from the history and from concurrent observation. Through deductive reasoning, we can reach a diagnosis because each item of information will fit within a previously established category. Suicidal ideation, hopelessness, and anorexia fall within the category of major depression but are sometimes found in other mental disorders as well. Adding early morning awakening, decreased energy, feelings of worthlessness, thoughts of guilt, impaired concentration, diurnal mood variation, and psychomotor retardation improves our confidence in making this diagnosis. In contrast to inductive problems, adding more items usually narrows the choice of the deductive answer.

In the inductive process, the unifying concept we need does not already exist, at least in the sense that a diagnostic category exists. We must create it. In other words, rather than matching the data to previously established categories, we try instead to create a category from the data available. It is an effort to synthesize the parts into a coherent whole.

Much of our training in clinical assessment focuses on deductive conclusions. We concentrate on diagnostic criteria, on indications for a particular treatment or course of action, on causes of behavior. We thus look for descriptive characteristics (early morning awakening), for decision points (suicidal ideation with a plan/without a plan), and for dynamic or other antecedents (early deprivation, abusive trauma). Much less of our training helps us think inductively. As a result, we may find the effort to think through a treatment plan unfamiliar and more difficult. To become more comfortable with the inductive process that underlies treatment planning, you may want to formalize the exercise with a series of questions. We have made use of some of these questions in earlier discussions.

To conceptualize the AIM, the questions that ask you to reach an inductive conclusion include the following:

1. What is the best possible outcome for therapy with this patient?
2. If this period of therapy succeeds to the greatest extent possible, how will this person's current life have changed for the better?

3. If, at the end of therapy, this person will have achieved the best possible solution to his or her current problems, what will that solution be?
4. How will this patient's life circumstances be as improved as possible if therapy can help him or her make the best use of inner resources, personal skills, and social situation?

These questions focus on the optimum outcome of the contemplated therapy, each from a slightly different perspective. Question 1 asks for the global result of therapy. Question 2 defines the issue in terms of a change in life circumstances. Question 3 introduces the concept of finding a "solution" to the presenting problems. Question 4 emphasizes the limits exerted by the patient's personal assets and liabilities. They are all variations of the core question: What should be the AIM of this therapy with this patient?

To illustrate how the inductive process might apply to a clinical problem, we can return to the case of Gary the Gay Gardener described earlier in this book.[3] In this brief example, only a few facts are available: Gary seeks therapy because of anxiety attacks and episodes of depersonalization. His symptoms developed over time as his long-term partner, Peter, continued his promiscuous behavior with other men. Gary loves Peter but is angry at his behavior, jealous of his attentions to other men, and fearful that Peter will contract AIDS. Although his psychological distress seems directly referable to Peter's behavior, we also know Gary is a gifted landscape designer who keeps his sexual preference a secret for fear of social and occupational consequences. How do these disparate clinical observations fit together? What concept underlies them?

We might first note the conflicting emotions Gary feels for Peter: on the one hand, affection and desire, but on the other, anger, jealousy, and fear. Identifying the single unifying concept, *emotions,* that contains these five affective states is an example of inductive logic. By recognizing that the emotions are in conflict, we add another level of abstraction, contained in the term *ambivalence.* In a similar way, we can abstract from Gary's desire to keep his sexual identity secret from his family and employer (although perhaps also reflecting a realistic fear of discrimination) that he is a man who avoids confrontation. Combining these two ideas leads to an initial hypothesis: Gary's ambivalent feelings toward Peter create inner turmoil that cannot be resolved because of his reluctance to confront Peter, and the unresolved turmoil fuels his episodes of anxiety

---

[3] See case vignette, Chapter 1, pages 1–2.

and depersonalization. This formulation now suggests that the AIM of therapy might be *resolution of ambivalence*. Would this result be the best single outcome? Yes, if it resolved the problem that brought Gary into therapy.

A similar set of questions may help focus on the GOALS that would bring about this desired result:

1. What must happen over the course of the therapy to bring about the chosen AIM?
2. Of what component problems does the AIM consist?
3. How can the issues revealed by the clinical assessment be grouped into meaningful categories?
4. What has to change in the patient's life circumstances, personality, maturity, coping ability, or other qualities for him or her to achieve the optimum outcome of the therapy?

These questions again look at the process of planning therapy GOALS from different viewpoints. Question 1 asks generally what must happen during therapy so that it achieves its desired result. Question 2 asks how the GOALS can be delineated as clearly defined problems. Question 3 asks for the abstract definition that will group items into a single category, much as our earlier example of fruits and chicken. Question 4 looks at those qualities of the patient whose improvement might contribute to the AIM. As with the AIM, these or similar questions prompt you to think inductively about what the therapy must accomplish.

Using question 4 to proceed with planning Gary's treatment, we might try two GOALS: clarify his relationship needs (to see whether Peter meets them and why) and empower confrontation (to help him deal more effectively with Peter's behavior). The first GOAL inductively moves from the observation of conflicted feelings to the more abstract concept that these feelings arise from aspects of the relationship between the two men, and it postulates that understanding these needs will foster resolution of conflicted feelings. The second GOAL simply reverses cause (avoidance of confrontation) with effect (unresolved tension between the men) on the assumption that successful confrontation will reduce that tension. Succeeding with both will, it is hoped, allow Gary to resolve the ambivalence, the chosen AIM of the therapy.

Sometimes it may be difficult to frame the GOALS in terms of the AIM you have first selected. Although this difficulty might indicate you are struggling with the inductive process, another possibility should also be considered. If the GOALS do not seem to point toward the proposed AIM, it can also mean the AIM should be reexamined. Perhaps it is overly broad or too narrow. Or it could be a poor fit with the clinical circumstances. The AIM may be inappropriate or unrealistic. How can you clarify these issues?

Suppose our formulation for Gary's case suggested that his troubles with Peter resulted in a "loss of self-esteem." In this instance, the inductive move to the abstract level results in an overgeneralization, encompassing more information than is found in the history, and illustrates how inductive logic may, when overly inclusive, be just as misleading as when it is too narrow. To carry this example forward: Although Gary may have lost some self-esteem, the loss is a secondary effect of his relationship troubles, and *self-esteem* is a vague term that might encompass narcissism, mood stability, and social position. This overly broad formulation would presumably suggest the AIM to be *increase self-esteem*. Finding appropriate therapy GOALS would reflect this ambiguity. Protect his narcissism? Gary might have suffered a narcissistic blow when Peter was unfaithful, but the therapy cannot control Peter's behavior. Raise his social standing? Therapy cannot do that either. Stabilize his mood? Gary is anxious, but neither depressed nor manic. An AIM based on an inaccurate formulation creates unhelpful GOALS and results in a poor treatment plan.

The clinical assessment provides the material for the formulation, and it is from the formulation that you must inductively derive the appropriate and realistic AIM. If you are unable to find the necessary GOALS for the AIM initially chosen, you may need to review and revise the formulation. Does it support the original AIM? Does it instead suggest that a different AIM would be a better fit with the patient's history and presentation? If the revised AIM is an improvement, finding the GOALS to support it will be easier.

Synthesizing a general concept from a group of historical facts, presenting complaints, and clinical observations is easier if you write them down and study the list, grouping items together and then finding similarities or contrasts among those groups.

I also recommend that therapists use written planning diagrams. A written diagram helps organize the treatment process and provides a concrete way to examine the course of therapy. It may be helpful during the necessary process of negotiating with the patient, and when completed, it should, like the treatment plan itself, reflect a consensus between therapist and patient on what they will try to do together. The diagram should be made a part of the patient's clinical record, where its presence will support third-party payment claims and provide required regulatory documentation. More important, the written record will help the therapist follow the plan worked out with the patient, especially if reviewed before and after each session. Case notes written after each session should also be organized to show what GOALS were worked on and what progress was made.

MOVING FROM ASSESSMENT TO FORMULATION

From the standpoint of treatment planning, the formulation must be a primary objective of the initial assessment.

Assessment often begins before we meet the patient. The referring source, which could be family, friends, a physician, or another mental health professional, provides us with significant information about the patient, the presenting problem, and even key features of the past history. As a result, we may approach the first interview with ideas, expectations, and half-formed plans that can help or hinder the assessment. Patients may also arrive with a set of expectations about psychotherapy, about what will be expected of them, and about us. If they have had prior contact with a psychotherapist, they are likely to be somewhat trained in the approach the earlier therapist favored. For example, patients who have seen a psychoanalytically oriented therapist may believe that the meeting will consist of their talking and the therapist passively listening or that they are expected to say anything that comes into their minds, rather than attempting to give an organized and coherent account of themselves and their difficulties.

The initial meeting with the patient is unique. The therapist's influence will probably never be as strong as during this initial contact. There is a certain "magical" quality with which therapist is invested, a projection of the patient's hopes and fears onto the blank screen that results from knowing very little about the therapist. The patient may project onto the therapist feelings, attitudes, and expectations carried over from earlier, perhaps unresolved, relationships. The patient's attitude may also reflect some reasonable hope of benefit and a realistic expectation that the therapist is an expert who may be able to help where family, friends, or coworkers could not.

A good relationship between therapist and patient is a highly significant factor in promoting a positive outcome for therapy (Luborsky and Auerbach 1985). A large part of it depends on the therapeutic alliance, or working alliance (Greenson 1967), that links the patient's motivation and intellectual appreciation of possible benefit with the therapist's presentation as an interested expert with a genuine desire to facilitate that benefit. A strong consensus accepts the therapeutic alliance as a central feature of all psychotherapies, regardless of orientation (Bateman 2002), and Meissner (1996) examined it in relation to both the real relationship with the therapist and the distortions introduced by transference and countertransference issues. In addition to the more realistic side of this beginning relationship, the patient's early positive attitude may engender a placebo effect (Goldstein 1960), as the hopefulness of an untried source of help translates into an ability to make forward progress. The patient may be ready to overcome some initial obstacles without any formal intervention by the therapist. This attitude can help build the initial rapport or, if unrealistic expectations are unmet, lead to disappointment and an unwarranted discouragement.

Therapists who recognize this early phenomenon can manage it better. They can allow it to promote the developing rapport if they simply proceed without comment, or they can diminish its influence by deliberately filling in some of the blanks. This injection of realism will not necessarily stifle hope; it may strengthen it if the patient recognizes the therapist's expertise and planfulness. The magical aspect will diminish in any case as over time the patient comes to know the therapist more realistically. It can also dramatically reappear as a more organized positive transference or be overshadowed by negative transference feelings. Either development may have to be dealt with if the therapy is to make further progress, but at the beginning, while it is there, this expectation and willingness can carry the therapy forward. The early match between the patient's expectations and the therapist's influence may account for the surprisingly strong early progress most patients make in therapy. Indeed, the reports of patients' improvement while on a waiting list (Endicott and Endicott 1963) or after a single session with the therapist—results that can represent permanent gains (Malan et al. 1975)—may be a consequence of this matchup.

As the initial interview progresses, the therapist will try to gain an increasingly clear and more meaningful idea of the patient's problems. The historical facts that emerge will be important in shaping this judgment. The therapist's impression of the patient's state of mind and mental capacities, as they are exhibited in the interview, is equally helpful, and the therapist may conduct a formal mental status examination in which, for example, cognitive skills such as memory, orientation, and reasoning are tested by a series of standardized questions. A great deal of information will emerge before this portion of the interview; it may even obviate it. Memory function, for instance, will show up in the ease and consistency with which the patient can provide historical data ranging from very recent to very distant events. A fair judgment of intelligence can be gained by appreciating the language the patient uses to describe his or her situation. Formal history taking has an influence on the therapist-patient relationship. Structured questioning, formal mental status testing, note taking during the interview, and especially separate testing procedures by written test or computer—all of these exact a price because they separate therapist and patient and create a more detached relationship. In certain cases—such as single-visit consultation for a court or agency or even a psychopharmacology consultation—this distancing may be appropriate and even helpful.

Active listening by the therapist centers on the process of making and testing hypotheses about the patient. From the earliest moment, we must generate ideas about the nature and causes of the patient's problems. We then listen to and observe the patient for information that will either support our hypothesis or disprove it and make way for another. Hypotheses are questions we hope to answer as patients tell us more about themselves. We generate a series of hypotheses to arrive at a diagnostic conclusion. We may initially consider a single episode of major depression; then revise it, on learning of prior depressions, to major depression, recurrent; and then revise it again to bipolar disorder if the history reveals an earlier episode of mania.

In addition to their utility in the important task of establishing the diagnosis, hypotheses are useful in planning the treatment. As we listen to the patient, we try to look behind the words, behind the phenomenology of the interview, to find the meaning of the patient's story. We form impressions about the patient's personality and motivation, and we look for the cause-and-effect relationship between the history the patient gives us and the presenting problems. We express these ideas as questions we pose to ourselves. The ideas may be quite simple. We may wonder, for example, if the patient is distorting the truth. Our hypothesis might be stated in this way: Is the patient exaggerating in an attempt to impress me? The ideas may be complex, as in the case of a patient whose history shows a pattern of job losses: Does this patient sabotage every job she takes in an effort to get back at her parents for not giving her everything she wanted and to convince her husband that he should take care of her?

These hypotheses are not necessarily ideas we want to share with the patient. Some therapists seem compelled to share every clever idea or newly created hypothesis, but the therapist who never has an unexpressed thought is a poor therapist indeed. Discretion is the better part of vanity. That being said, we can help our assessment along if we selectively test out some of our hypotheses during the interview. Often we can resolve a question by presenting it, at the appropriate moment, to the patient and asking for his or her response. We can simply tell the patient our thoughts and invite comment. We can offer a cautious interpretation and try to judge by the response whether our idea is a valid one.

Judging the results of presenting an interpretation is always tricky. The patient may agree, perhaps with a simple "Yes, you're right," and yet leave us unconvinced. The patient may disagree but with such a strong denial that we suspect the answer may really be yes. Perhaps the most revealing response to an interpretation, whether the initial answer is yes or no, is when it provokes new, relevant material about the issue we have raised. As an example, consider again the case of Ernest the Edgy Engineer.[4] His wife found him with a shotgun and shells, and she worried that he was about to shoot himself. In the initial interview, we say, "Sitting there with the shotgun must have been a temptation. All your troubles would be over and you wouldn't have to suffer." Although this is a superficial "interpretation," it does ask two implied questions: Was he planning to shoot himself? Does he concern himself with the effect such an action would have on others?

Ernest answers, "I was just cleaning it. My son and I were going hunting. I always clean my guns before I go." He denies a suicidal "temptation." Should we believe him?

He then goes on to say, "Besides, I knew a guy once who did that. Blew off his whole head. Had to bury him in a closed casket. And he had less problems than me, as far as I could tell. Seemed to be doing just fine and then one day, boom." After the denial comes a memory with worrisome overtones. There is narcissistic concern about how he would look after a shotgun blast, an association less reassuring than if he had thought about its effect on family members. There is the implication that his explanation of cleaning the gun, like the bland façade of the man he remembers, is no guarantee of his safety. The memory suggests a possible inclination to identify with and imitate the other man. All in all, Ernest's indirect response tells us his explanation of cleaning the gun merits careful further investigation.

During the assessment period, whether it occupies one interview or extends over several, we will concentrate on getting the history from the patient. Our history taking can fall within a continuum. At one end we can adopt a totally unstructured approach, in which the patient chooses what to say, guided by only the most open-ended of questions from the therapist. At the other end we can structure the interview completely and ask a series of predetermined questions designed to "fill in the blanks" in

---

[4]See case vignette, Chapter 2, pages 19–20.

an exhaustive outline, with the patient speaking only in answer to our questions. Some computer-based histories follow this pattern, but so do some interviewers. Both extreme approaches have their place. An unstructured approach might be useful in an assessment for classical psychoanalysis, where the analyst wants to elicit material unbiased by his or her own interests and to see how well the prospective analysand can do with a neutral, passive listener. A completely structured approach might be helpful in a research design in which the protocol requires a full set of data to enhance the validity of the study. For our purposes, however, neither extreme is useful, and both could actually impair our treatment planning.

Most of us, during the period we were in training, took exhaustive histories in which we tried to document and understand everything of significance in the patient's life from birth to the present. Sometimes we included events prior to birth as we explored the entire genealogy of the patient and constructed a family tree. In attempting to fulfill this training exercise, completeness seemed more important than relevance. In clinical practice, however, the attempt to gather every possible historical fact, relevant or irrelevant, diffuses the interviewer's focus and makes it more difficult to decide what issues are truly important. An exhaustive, unfocused approach may damage the therapist-patient relationship. Half a dozen interviews, extending over as many weeks, might get every fact about the patient surveyed and recorded, but meanwhile, the patient must tolerate the mental pain and ongoing crisis that provoked the referral, and rapport suffers.

We do not need to know everything there is to know about someone to provide an effective treatment plan. If we concentrate on the important issues—and usually this means the issues important to the patient—we will have in hand the most useful information we can get at the time. We can be confident that other historical information of importance will emerge in due course and at a time when its significance may be more easily appreciated. In the same way, we can rely on the eventual emergence of material of significance to the presenting problem, including such factors as unresolved developmental issues, poorly integrated traumas, or unsolved crises. They can determine the shape and form of the patient's presentation; they may even lie behind the immediate crisis and yet not always be apparent during the initial interview.

At some point in the interview, the therapist will have decided on a formal diagnosis. More experienced interviewers accumulate the necessary data for this decision without making diagnosis their primary focus (Guaron and Dickinson 1966). Some interesting studies show that a diagnostic conclusion may be reached very early in the interview, even within the first 3 minutes (Sandifer et al. 1970). These early judgments are not infallible; later data may suggest different answers. The less experienced interviewer may need more time for diagnostic decision making.

Efforts to improve diagnostic certainty use new information and new methodology. Better technology provides us with more knowledge of the biological and environmental determinants of mental disorders. The use of standardized diagnostic instruments helps to clarify areas of uncertainty, such as dissociative disorders (Bremner et al. 1993) and personality disorders (Gunderson et al. 1994). Clinical field trials use structured interviews to assess individual diagnoses (Williams et al. 1992), to measure overall diagnostic agreement (Robins et al. 1988), and to establish interrater reliability on diagnosis (Regier et al. 1994) on an international scale. New theoretical approaches, such as "decision analysis," seek to decrease uncertainty in diagnostic reasoning (Zarin and Earls 1993). All of this progress means that an accurate diagnosis becomes increasingly important in patient assessment. We must recognize especially those conditions for which a specific treatment is indicated. Mood disorders, the psychoses, some anxiety disorders, and even some seemingly learned habit patterns have been shown to respond to an increasingly sophisticated pharmacological armamentarium. The correct diagnosis will help us select the optimal treatment STRATEGY and TACTICS for a particular patient.

Important as the diagnosis may be, however, treatment planning is a critical task as well. The initial interview must provide not only a diagnosis but also the kind of information that will more clearly help us determine the AIM of the therapy, and it must provide the kind of relevant data that will serve as a rational basis for choosing its GOALS. The sooner we can form an adequate diagnostic impression, the more of the interview's valuable time we can use to lay the foundation for a solid, workable treatment plan.

THREE QUESTIONS FOR PLANNING

In addition to obtaining the obvious historical material—the chief complaint, present and past history, family history, and so on—we should be able, at the end of the first interview, to answer three important questions.

Question 1: Why Did the Patient Come HERE?

This question seeks more information than who sent the patient, how the appointment was made, and how the patient chose us from among the many practitioners available—the mechanics of the referral. It also asks why the patient specifically selected a mental health provider. Although the answer might seem obvious, it may not be as clear as it first looks. In the Epidemiologic Catchment Area study (Regier et al. 1993), it was found that nearly three-quarters of all people in the United States with a diagnosable mental or addictive disorder did not seek help for it. Of the remaining quarter, more went to general medical specialists or other sources than to specialists in mental and addictive disorders. This study showed that less than half (40.5%) of the visits made by those who did seek help were visits to a mental health specialist (Narrow et al. 1993). What these figures tell us is that those few patients who want help look for it less often from a mental health specialist than from anyone else. One reason is the continuing stigma attached to mental disorders. Another is the reluctance to admit to some kind of mental "weakness." Self-reliance and cultural expectations support alternatives like prayer, hard work, willpower, or other self-generated efforts. Many sources of help are available in place of the mental health professional, such as self-help programs modeled on the 12-step format of Alcoholics Anonymous: Overeaters Anonymous, Narcotics Anonymous, Gamblers Anonymous, and so on. Not only do mental health professionals play no role in these organizations but their participation is actively excluded to avoid additional stigma and to create an atmosphere of peer-generated assistance. To avail themselves of a mental health resource, then, patients must decide first to acknowledge their difficulties and "publicly" seek outside help; second, to choose a professional source of help over one of the many self-help avenues; and third, to select a mental health professional over other professional sources of help. Such a patient is a distinctly unusual member of a small minority.

Why did this person come **here?** asks how this choice came about. What elements of their problem do patients define as mental illness? What allows them to overcome the stigma and the resulting reluctance to acknowledge such a problem? What makes them choose professional help over a less stigmatizing (and perhaps less expensive) source of assistance? And what brings them specifically to a mental health professional rather than to one of the other sources of professional help? As we explore these questions, we will better understand why our patient falls into that select group of those who both seek and find mental health care. We will be able to identify more fully what expectations the patient includes in that choice and to define the patient's needs more clearly.

Although many patients are referred, others pick a name out of the telephone book. These patients have not asked a friend, a family physician, or a member of the clergy to recommend a mental health professional. Are they too ashamed to confide their intentions, even as they feel they must seek some kind of help? Are they so isolated from others that they do not know anyone to trust with this sensitive question? Are they somewhat "paranoid" about their need for help and want to keep it secret? Again, our question *Why here?* can help us sort out the answers.

Patients who decide they need professional mental health services rather than self-help services may believe their problems are more serious than a self-help organization, composed of other people like themselves, could manage. They may feel "crazy," about to lose control, fated for a deteriorating course. Determining why they came *here* helps to uncover such covert questions.

Another example: Patients sometimes go to their family doctor with vague physical symptoms in the belief that they are ill with some undefined medical disorder. The doctor takes a history, examines them, and obtains the results of a battery of laboratory tests but is unable to document a specific medical illness. Noting some evidence that the person is under "stress," the doctor suggests a mental health referral and sends the patient along to you. What the patient may have heard is that the doctor thinks the problem "is all in my head," meaning that it is trivial or even imaginary. This person may want you to contradict that perceived negative judgment and to find that the problem is a physical illness after all. As a result, until that expectation is met or modified by discussion, the patient is not going to be receptive to a proposal for psychotherapy, because it would only confirm the belief that the problem is being misdiagnosed and overlooked. This person has come to your office to obtain your expert rebuttal of the doctor's apparent dismissal of his or her complaints.

The answer to *Why did this person come* **here?** must be more than an understanding of the mechanics of the referral, more than the fact that your name is in the Yellow Pages, more than the knowledge that a local physician thought you could be of help. A careful exploration of the motives behind the mechanics can help you clarify and understand the request for treatment and the patient's suitability for it.

Question 2: Why Did the Patient Come NOW?

Most of the time, a problem for which someone seeks your help is of long standing. It may have existed for months or years without bringing him or her to the point of asking for professional help. We want to know why this person came to see you at this *particular* moment in time. Why not last week, last month, a year ago? Why not next month, or later still, or even not at all? We are asking, then, what precipitated this request for treatment.

When a problem is long-standing, the sufferer develops a tolerance for it that creates a kind of inertia, a tendency to put up with difficulties whose cost, in terms of limitations or distress, is still bearable. Whatever the precipitant that brings the patient to your office might be, it must be strong enough to overcome this inertia and the reluctance that person feels about seeking help. This reluctance may be simple embarrassment or shame about having a mental disorder; it might indicate a desire not to reveal fears, fantasies, inner feelings, hopes, and dreams; it might be self-consciousness, fear of ridicule, or guilt. A precipitating event or influence sufficient to overcome these barriers must be a very important one indeed. If we understand it fully, we will know what problem or what aspect of the problem is most important to our patient. That knowledge improves our chance of proposing a treatment plan that is clearly related to this most important issue, and it will help identify the problem area the patient will work most diligently with us to correct.

Question 3: What Does the Patient WANT?

Remember the old joke in which the interviewer asks, "Now, Mr. Jones, what brought you to the hospital?" and the patient answers sincerely, "I came on a bus"? The better question is "Mr. Jones, what do you want your hospital visit to accomplish?"

Our third question is the most important. A workable treatment plan must take into account not only what the therapist can do for the patient but also what it is the patient wants done. Through discussion and ultimately negotiation, patient and therapist must arrive at an agreement as to what they hope will be the outcome of the therapy and how they will work together to see that they attain it. To initiate this negotiated part of the treatment plan, the therapist will need a clear and comprehensive idea of what the patient wants. Only when the patient's request for help can be understood will the therapist know whether to try to provide the requested service.

What the patient *wants* includes a wide spectrum of requests. In one survey (Frank et al. 1978), patients' wants ranged from the mundane (administrative help, clarification, advice) to the sophisticated (psychodynamic insight, psychological expertise) and from the more open (ventilation, reality contact, nonpsychiatric medical treatment) to the more covert (control, succor, confession). Some wanted "nothing"; they were referred through misunderstanding or mistake or at the insistence of others. The answer to the question of what the patient wants must be as concrete and as detailed as possible. It is not sufficient to know the patient wants to be "happy" or wants relief of symptoms. We need to know what that person means by "happiness" and which symptoms he or she wants resolved.

For example, suppose a man comes in distraught over his wife's decision to divorce him. He suspects she is seeing another man but does not know who, although he thinks it might be her boss. He loves his wife and is unwilling to let her go. The stress of her plan to file the divorce papers has kept him from sleeping, destroyed his concentration, and saddled him with persistent pounding headaches. What does he want? He might want us to talk her out of it. We would be unlikely to succeed, even if she agreed to come in with him. Certainly he and I cannot hope, sitting in the office without her, to do anything about her decision. He might instead want us to see her and find out the identity of the other man. This role, gathering information for the patient, would probably be unacceptable, because it might well involve some deception in our dealings with the patient's wife. Perhaps all he wants is to get some pills to help him sleep and take away the headaches. We would probably not agree to merely supply medication for symptomatic relief. Alternatively, he might want us to help him let go of his wife, to see him through the crisis, and work with him as he goes through the divorce. That sounds more like it. We might be able to help him with that request.

The answer to this third question should also provide us with some idea of how the patient expects to get help from us and to participate in that help. Some patients might believe that if they say everything that is on their mind, the therapist will provide the answers they want. Other patients, who want "insight" without realizing they must use that insight to change their behavior, are in trouble before the therapy starts. Still others might feel they must do all the work while the therapist sits by as a benign but interested observer. Finally, some patients may want to take the opposite tack and expect the therapist to do all the work.

What patients want may not be entirely clear from their verbal statements. Covert needs must be surmised from body language, historical clues, or "reading between the lines." Once understood, covert needs may be raised with the patient, as part of the assessment process, to confirm or eliminate the suspected issue. When the therapist understands what the patient wants, he or she can agree or can try to modify the request. The effort to clarify the patient's requests will usually be the first piece of therapeutic work patient and therapist will accomplish together. As such, its success or failure will shape the manner in which they work together afterward.

The assessment process involves much more than the answers to these three questions, important as they are. The answers must be combined with the history and with the therapist's appreciation of the mental state and the abilities of the person sitting across the room. The therapist must make a global judgment about the patient's capacity to use therapy and about what general type of therapy will provide the best fit. Patients vary in age, maturity, intelligence, suggestibility, empathy, and verbal skills, as well as in their ability to relate to others, their openness for change, their tolerance of anxiety, and the severity of their psychological deficits. These and other variables will determine how well the patient can engage with a particular therapeutic modality; the qualities that select for psychodynamic psychotherapy, for example, differ from those for behavior modification. These factors determine where the patient falls along what is usually referred to as the expressive-supportive continuum (Winston et al. 1986). Patients at the expressive end may be better suited for intrapsychic, insight-oriented therapies that seek to change personality structure. They can respond to a therapist who remains neutral, declines to gratify their needs, and reveals as little personal data as possible. Patients at the supportive end may be better suited for interpersonal approaches designed to support or reestablish their emotional status quo. They respond better to an actively engaging therapist who selectively gratifies their needs and who is appropriately self-disclosing. Most patients will fall somewhere in the middle of these two extremes.

Integrating all of this material provides a sound basis for arriving at a formulation summarizing and explaining the patient's current dilemma and the paths that led to it, a formulation that lays the foundation for the design of a useful treatment plan. A sample initial interview can illustrate how the assessment process might work.

ASSESSMENT FOR PLANNING

Alice the Anxious Actress

My new supervisee, Arthur, is a psychiatry resident starting the second half of his outpatient psychotherapy rotation. I have arranged to sit in on one of his initial interviews. In the waiting room, he greets Alice, a slender woman with long hair, wearing a shape-hugging rust-brown dress buttoned up to her neck, who looks about her stated age, 28. She responds to Arthur with a nervous smile and accepts his explanation of my presence. I say hello to her and notice a slight tremor when she extends her hand. Her grip is loose and her palm is a little moist. We enter the interview room, and I take a seat at the far side, out of their line of sight.

I have already formed a tentative diagnosis. I think Alice has an anxiety syndrome. It could be generalized, situational, or phobic—perhaps a social phobia. I do not think she is psychotic or significantly depressed. All this has been formed when hardly three words have been spoken, and I have based this early impression on observations I make automatically: She makes good eye contact; her voice, facial expression, and posture suggest anxiety but not a depressed mood or an elated one; her tremor and moist grip add to my impression and also raise the added question of an overactive thyroid. I am clearly making a lot out of very little real data, perhaps too much. Her anxiety could be either her response to the novelty of the interview or her reason for seeking help from the clinic, and her diagnosis could turn out, with more information, to be something else entirely. I mention my early idea for two reasons. First, I am thinking of the diagnosis from the first moment of the interview. Second, I may be able to reach the conclusion I need quite quickly, and if so, I can direct my energy in the interview toward whether treatment is needed and how to plan it.

Arthur begins by asking her, "What brings you to the clinic?" I make a mental note to discuss that with him afterward. My opening question would be "What can I do for you?" I want to find the answers to my three assessment questions as soon as I can. My opening question asks, in effect, *What does she want?*

"I always feel nervous," Alice says. "It's like I have stage fright all the time." These statements support my idea about generalized anxiety, but the reference to stage fright keeps social phobia as a possibility, too. Arthur begins taking a history. To summarize what she tells us: Alice is trying to pursue an acting career while supporting herself working as a sales clerk. Last year she got a small part in a play being staged by a local repertory group and began dating Adam, one of the actors. Soon Adam was suggesting they get married; he had offered her an engagement ring, but Alice put him off. She liked him, but she was not sure it would work, worried they would not earn enough between them. Her own parents had been poor and were now divorced, and she did not want to repeat their experience.

Arthur spends the next few minutes finding out about her presenting symptom, "feeling nervous." She tells him she was always high strung but the last year or so has been worse. She feels tense and apprehensive almost all the time and has lost a little weight, although she does not think she is eating less than usual. She sleeps all right, but sometimes it takes her a long time to fall asleep. Once in a while she is awakened by nightmares, although she does not remember what is in them. Her nervousness is worse when she is around other people. At work she is more comfortable with the customers than socializing with her coworkers on a break.

At this point I have four hypotheses. One: she is mildly avoidant and socially phobic, with symptoms gradually worsening as she takes on more responsibility. Two: her anxiety reflects unresolved family issues, probably related to her parents' divorce. Three: she has been unable to break off her relationship with Adam even though she finds something about it threatening; the threat, real or not, produces situational anxiety. Four: her apparent anxiety could be a symptom of an overactive thyroid. I could add a fifth possibility: her sleep and appetite disturbances raise the possibility that she is depressed. Yet her insomnia is initial, not terminal, and her loss of appetite is consistent with anxiety as well as depression. Moreover, she does not look depressed, and so far these mild neurovegetative signs are the only indicators of a possible mood disorder. If I were doing the interview, I would focus my history taking on areas that might clarify these possibilities. Because I am only an observer, I am limited to listening for evidence for or against them, and for now I do not think depression is very likely. Note that these are not the only hypotheses I could come up with, but they are the ones that most closely match what I know so far. In thinking about these cause-and-effect issues during the interview, I have already begun to formulate the case.

Arthur now asks Alice about her family and learns her parents were divorced when she was 11, although she remembers them fighting for years before that. She and her younger brother were sent to stay with a maternal aunt. Those 2 years were a happier time and a relief from the tension in her parents' home. Her mother remarried, and they returned to live with her. Alice's stepfather was a well-to-do businessman who could afford to send her to college. After she graduated, she found a job and began taking acting classes.

This history strengthens my "family issues" hypothesis, and I am less inclined toward the idea of a social phobia. The stress of her relationship with Adam, on top of her history of disrupted parenting, points toward a more specific etiology.

Arthur now asks a series of specific questions about her early childhood development and about her health. None of these routine questions yields any useful information. He then does a brief mental status examination. Her cognitive functions and judgment are intact. She denies feelings of hopelessness, helplessness, or suicidal thoughts. She denies hallucinations and delusions. Arthur does not learn more from his formal exam than he might have surmised from her general presentation in the interview.

He inquires about any prior episodes of anxiety. He ascertains that she has not had panic episodes, that her anxiety has made it harder to concentrate on her work, and that she has been more irritable than usual and often has a headache at the end of the day. She is sometimes anxious even in comfortable situations—for example, she says, when she is spending time with Adam. Arthur goes on to ask her about her school experiences and learns that she was a popular and outgoing girl who had some success acting in class plays and a local theater group. These successes convinced her to try for a stage career. I now discard the social phobia hypothesis, despite the possibility that her acting efforts were early counterphobic defenses to overcome a constitutional shyness. I wish Arthur would stop delving into the past and would spend more time on her current relationship with her boyfriend. Finally he gets back to it, and Alice tells him Adam is a warm and thoughtful person who seems genuinely interested in taking care of her. Their sexual relationship, she says, has been satisfying.

I notice, however, that her voice trembles a bit, and there is a slight frown in her expression. Arthur either does not notice this change or chooses to ignore it. Alice goes on to say that she knows Adam loves her, and she thinks she loves him, but she is not sure. Arthur asks if her worry about their finances is the only problem she has about accepting his proposal. Alice says it is but looks uncomfortable, and I sense she is concerned about something else that she is so far unwilling to reveal. Arthur does not pursue the possible "secret" but instead changes the subject. He asks her about her sales job and about her efforts to pursue an acting career. Her answers do not add anything to my effort to understand her anxiety. At this point we are near the end of the interview hour, and Arthur turns to me to ask if I might have any questions for her.

"Yes," I say, "I was wondering how you happened to choose the clinic for help with this problem." In other words: Why did you come here?

"I don't have much money," Alice tells me, "and when my doctor couldn't find anything wrong, he said I should try counseling for my nervousness."

"Did he do a thyroid test, do you know?"

"Yes, he did. It was normal."

"Did he give you any medication for the nervousness?"

"He offered to. I said I didn't want to depend on a pill."

If Alice came to us out of economic necessity, I wonder (to myself) whether she might feel she was settling for a lower quality of care. That bias might influence her ability to accept and to participate in the treatment we recommend. The family doctor suspected a thyroid problem, too, and it appears that he ruled it out. I learn that Alice has rejected medication as a "solution" to her anxiety. I go on to my next assessment question: Why now?

"Alice, you've had this problem with your nerves for about a year. Why did you decide to get some help for it at this point?"

"Things just kept getting worse. I guess I was tired of putting up with it."

"Yes, but what made you finally decide? What was the last straw?"

"Oh. Well, now that you remind me, it was when Adam started pressuring me about our getting married. I thought to myself, 'I'm not well enough to do that,' and I said that to him. And he said I have to get some help with it, so I went to my doctor the next day."

Alice's answer raises new questions. How strong is the secondary gain of being "sick"? It protects her by allowing her to defer the decision about marriage without agreeing to something she is unsure about or risking Adam's anger and the possible loss of his involvement. How much will this factor undermine her ability to profit from therapy? By not accepting her first, rather vague, response to my question, "Why now?" I have elicited an important factor to consider in later treatment planning. The hour is winding up. I ask my final question.

"Now that you're here, I wonder what kind of help you think would be best for your problem. Your doctor wanted to give you medication. What do you think would be helpful?"

"I thought I should try talking with somebody about my problem," Alice answers. "Sort of, you know, two heads are better than one."

Again I try to get a more precise, more helpful, answer. "And how do you see that helping you get over the anxiety problem? What do you think will happen when you talk about the problem with a therapist?"

Alice looks puzzled. "I don't know, exactly. Maybe I can get some suggestions about what to do. I don't know."

"We're almost out of time. The last thing I wanted to ask you is what you expect the therapy to do for you. What do you hope will be better at the end of it if everything works out for you?"

"You're asking some hard questions." Alice thinks for a moment. "I guess two things. I don't want to be nervous all the time. And I want to figure out what to do about Adam. Should I marry him or not? I'm all confused about that."

"I know what you mean," I say. "Marriage is a tough decision. Still, lots of people make it every day without coming to a therapist for help. Maybe they get advice from their friends and the family, but you're saying you need more than that. How come?"

I notice Alice's eyes grow moist, and she hesitates before answering. "I guess I'm just too screwed up to make it on my own," she says finally. "Don't you think you can help me?"

"I think we can. What we need to figure out with you is what's the best way to help and what we want the therapy to do."

Our time was up, and Arthur set up another appointment with Alice before she left. Arthur and I briefly discuss the interview. Alice's answers show she is unclear about how therapy could benefit her. She expects that the therapist, the expert, will tell her what to do. She does not at this point anticipate an active role for herself, though she is clear about what benefits she wants: symptomatic relief and the resolution of her dilemma about marrying Adam. Although these are relatively concrete requests, they are not unrealistic, and they can serve as a good starting point for designing her treatment plan, but first we need a formulation. The process by which we generate it can be divided into four steps: identification, exploration and clarification, setting hypotheses, and validation.

Before we return to Alice's case, we must lay out these four steps.

Step 1: Identification

The first step is to identify a significant problem or theme. Often patients will tell us what problems are significant, but we can also generate a problem list by actively listening to patients describe why they came here and why they came now. In a sense, we define a problem by comparing what patients say and do, and what kinds of issues are important to them, with normative standards. These standards are of two types: those patients apply to themselves and those the social group and the larger society apply to everybody.

Take Pablo again.[5] For a long while, he considered his pursuit of women to be an ego-boosting activity. Success made him feel good. Meanwhile, the larger society—in the form of his family and friends—looked on his activity as undesirable. He was breaching the norm of finding a mate, and some thought he was treating women badly, as sexual objects rather than as individuals. Later Pablo redefined his own norms and decided he was failing to reach a wider objective of his own. He might have characterized this objective as settling down and raising a family, for instance, or simply felt that he was tired of the seemingly endless string of romantic failures, when each infatuation failed to become an intimate relationship. If Pablo had not defined his pursuit of women as a problem, of course, we might never have encountered him as a patient. If we did encounter him because his family and friends, on the basis of their group norms, had pushed him into seeking an appointment, we would confront a patient whose hidden agenda might be to have us support his norms over those of the wider group. Still, patients are generally aware of societal norms, whether they agree with them or not, and they will often acknowledge a problem if we define it for them.

Once we have a workable idea about a problem area, we can either tell the patient about it or keep it to ourselves until we are more certain of our grounds. On the one hand, telling patients early provides an opportunity to hear whether they agree. Even a contradiction is helpful: Either it will convincingly rule out an issue we might otherwise pursue fruitlessly or it will stimulate us to make further efforts at understanding. On the other hand, not immediately telling patients what problems we have identified allows us to hear more about the issues without placing them on the defensive, possibly distorting or dissembling in an effort to persuade us otherwise. In any case, the original identification of a problem must be a tentative one. We often have an incomplete picture of the issue at that stage, and it is likely that we will need to revise it later. This leads us to the next step in our pursuit of a formulation.

Step 2: Exploration and Clarification

The second step is to explore and clarify the problems we have tentatively defined. The more we know about them, the more likely we are to draw the correct inferences. We want to explore each problem in sufficient depth to clarify its relationship to the patient's past and present mental health.

---

[5]See case vignette, Chapter 3, page 35.

A good part of this effort at clarification is phenomenological. Like a good newspaper reporter, we try to get the story, its who, what, when, where, why, and how. Who exactly were the women Pablo pursued? What were they like? Were there any similarities, any characteristics they shared? What were the differences between them? When was he first attracted to them? When did he start this pattern of pursuit? Where did he meet them? Where did he take them for dates? For sexual privacy? How did he approach them? How did he carry out his plan of conquest? We would continue to gather this phenomenological information from Pablo until we felt we had a reasonably clear picture of the activity that had brought him to see us.

An equally important part of our exploration concerns the context of behavior. We want to know the historical background and the frame of reference in which the identified problem occurs. What led up to it? What contemporary conditions allowed it to flourish? As we talk with Pablo and hear more about his involvement with the series of women, we listen for connections with earlier periods of his life. When did he begin to search for women in this way? How did his early conquests differ from the later ones? Why have the most recent experiences apparently been the least satisfactory? We will listen, too, for how his current compulsive womanizing affects other important areas of his life. How, for example, does it fit in with his work as an artist? Does it energize his artistic imagination, or does it distract him and undermine his creative efforts? Phenomenology and context allow us to define the problem in a variety of useful ways. Behavioral: What are the antecedents and the consequences of the behavior? Social: Within what systems does it function? Psychodynamic: What is its motivational and conflictual basis?

Although we identify problems and collect data about them in pursuit of the formulation, it is at this point, unfortunately, that some therapists may stop thinking. Instead of making active use of this excellent material, they may simply be satisfied that they "understand" the patient because they have assembled a coherent history. That is clearly not enough. We have the "what" part of the story but not the "why." To progress toward a useful formulation, we must put as much energy into understanding why the problem is there as we have in putting together a complete picture of what it is.

Step 3: Setting Hypotheses

The formulation, with its cause-and-effect account of the patient's presentation, uses the history and our observations to generate preliminary explanations, or hypotheses, which are the intermediate step between clinical assessment and final synthesis. Our third step, then, is to create one or more of these hypotheses, using these assessment materials to explain the patient's behavior, affects, and symptoms. We want to understand the importance of a particular problem in the patient's life and determine its significance. What does it gain for the patient? What are the costs paid for these gains? What does this behavior protect against? What is its importance intrapsychically? Interpersonally? Within the social framework? Our hypothesis may be complete, or it may be partial. A complete hypothesis explains not only the meaning of the behavior within the patient's current life but also its source in earlier experience and the multiple layers it may contain. A partial hypothesis more modestly tries to explain the facts as given by the patient so far. Both are important.

Constructing a complete hypothesis introduces a higher likelihood of error. We usually lack sufficient data at this early stage to evaluate its validity. We may surmise, for example, that Pablo pursues women in a compulsive repetition of his earlier relationship with his mother and father. Or we might think that his pursuit of the ideal woman is a way of avoiding long-term involvement with any woman. Perhaps we might wonder whether Pablo's Don Juan approach conceals an attraction to men he does not wish to acknowledge. None of these ideas can be confirmed or ruled out until we know a lot more about him than we do now.

A partial hypothesis should be easier to verify. Suppose Pablo has told us his most recent relationship was with Penny, a woman who reminded him of his mother: She encouraged him in his art to the point of seeming to take over his career. She was uncritical in her judgments of his work, lauding the bad with as much enthusiasm as the good, and he was attracted to her because she seemed such a fan, because he liked her praise and support. Why, then, did he break off the relationship? He felt smothered by her adulation, he tells us. He thought she was living through his efforts, and that he was being used. Pablo's statements might lead us to conclude he is struggling for emotional and professional independence from his mother and is playing this struggle out through surrogate mothers in the women he meets. We do not at this point know why he is doing so. We will need to hear more about both his relationship with his mother and those with other women before we can feel confident in this idea, but at least we have a hypothesis grounded in the facts we have gathered so far, rather than an idea plucked in its entirety from the pages of a book of theory.

Step 4: Validation

The final step is to test the hypotheses we think most likely to be valid. If possible, we want to confirm or rule them out before we make use of them for treatment planning. One way to investigate a hypothesis is to gather further information and to see whether that information supports or undermines our conclusion.

Our hypothesis that Penny, Pablo's recent love relationship, originally attracted him because she was supportive and encouraging like his mother provides an example. Suppose we ask Pablo whether there were any ways that she was not like his mother. He might tell us, yes, that Penny was a museum curator who knew a good deal about modern painting, whereas his mother had no formal training in art; in fact, his mother has what Pablo considers bad taste. Perhaps he would say further that Penny often criticized him for things he did, such as his habit of leaving his clothes all over the floor, whereas his mother had tolerated his sloppiness with a "boys will be boys" attitude…and so on. Contradictory information by itself, of course, would not rule out our hypothesis. It might be argued that Pablo had selected a woman who had just enough difference from his mother to keep this uncomfortable idea out of conscious awareness. However, the additional information clearly fills out the picture we have of Pablo's relationship with Penny. We might go on to explore it in even greater depth, with each additional piece of information modifying, confirming, or contradicting our original idea until we felt reasonably certain it was a valid starting point for understanding our patient.

Another way to evaluate a hypothesis is to test it in the consultation interview. Often this test might be in the form of an interpretation of some kind. Unlike an interpretation within a therapy context, a test interpretation is a one-time intervention, designed to elicit a response that will confirm or deny the underlying hypothesis. With Pablo, for example, we might choose to comment to him that the more Penny seemed to act like his mother, the less he liked her. Certainly this suggestion is not a very deep interpretation, nor should it be, but it does contain the idea that Pablo's feelings about his mother play a role in his comfort with another woman. The type of confirmation we would look for can occur at several levels. At the simplest level, the patient might simply agree. If Pablo said, "Yes, that's true," and changed the subject or stopped without having anything else to say, we might take his comment as positive, although weak, support. Better would be not only agreement but further material, stimulated by our remark and supporting the idea. Pablo might add to his acknowledgment, for instance, that Penny looked a little like his mother, or that both women had a habit of tilting their head to the side when they smiled. Better still, from the standpoint of supporting this hypothesis, would be the emergence of some new idea linked to its central premise. Pablo might go on to say that when his father met Penny, he had also remarked on her resemblance to Pablo's mother and that he, Pablo, had felt rather annoyed and upset with his father for making that remark. In therapy, such a new avenue might be pursued throughout the remainder of the session and perhaps beyond, but for the purposes of the evaluation it need go no further.

It is also possible to test the hypothesis by proposing it in the negative. The so-called null hypothesis may be easier to evaluate because, by definition, a single contradiction will invalidate it. If we use our same example, the null hypothesis would be this: Pablo's unsatisfactory relationships with women are not influenced or caused by his relationship with his mother. Given what we have already said about Pablo, Penny, and his mother, this particular null hypothesis would fall quickly. Consider, however, a more subtle example: the null hypothesis that Pablo's choice of a career in fine arts was not determined by insecurity with women. Does he, in other words, use his position as an artist to attract and interest women? We might ask Pablo whether he meets the women he gets involved with by employing them as models or through art shows or gallery exhibits. "No," he might say, "I don't. I don't use live models, and I've never met any of my dates at a gallery or art show. In fact, I try to avoid those affairs. They're all a bunch of phonies anyway." So, for now at least, we have no contradictory data, and this null hypothesis would stand.

All of these examples fall within the category of psychodynamic hypotheses. There are other categories as well: descriptive diagnosis, biological hypotheses, cognitive-behavioral hypotheses, and systems hypotheses (Frances et al. 1984). The diagnosis itself is a kind of hypothesis. It organizes a group of observations—the signs and symptoms—under a single heading that may have some predictive significance. The possibility that physical illness may present with an emotional or behavioral manifestation will lead to medical hypotheses. The medical condition of the patient provides another hypothesis-generating engine. Some psychiatric disorders have a more evident biological basis than others: bipolar disorder, some of the anxiety syndromes, and the organic psychoses are obvious examples. It is likely that even with the advances in molecular biology and the research associated with it, some psychiatric conditions—at least as currently defined—will remain behavioral rather than biological. Their etiology will be learned experiences that are unadaptive to contemporary conditions. The dissociative disorders and perhaps posttraumatic stress syndromes may fall under this heading. A biological hypothesis points toward a particular kind of treatment approach, one that often combines psychotherapy with a medical treatment. Cognitive-behavioral hypotheses delineate the current problem areas in terms of the antecedent events that provoke them and the responses that reinforce them. On what contingent factors does the problem behavior hinge, and what contingent results keep it going? Finally, systems hypotheses reflect the patient's place within social groups. Stresses within the family, the community, or a more inclusive system may provoke the observed problem. Sometimes the patient's problem behavior expresses a group norm, as when a delinquent adolescent acts out the conflicts within a dysfunctional family.

To the extent we share our hypotheses with the patient, we gain another prospective benefit. The patient sees we are making an active effort to understand him or her as a person, and if the relevance of our ideas resonates with the patient's expectation of help, that recognition of being understood strengthens the therapeutic alliance.

Clinical Example: Alice the Anxious Actress

As a final example of formulating a case, let us return to my supervisee's assessment of the young actress with the anxiety symptoms from earlier in this chapter.

Arthur calls me to say that Alice telephoned him the day after our joint meeting to ask whether I could come to the second interview. Arthur adds that he would like it, too. The training program rarely provides direct demonstrations by the attendings, and it would be a chance for him to see the way I work. I think Arthur is right. The residents need to see how experienced psychiatrists work, much the way our surgical colleagues bring their residents into the operating room. I agree to return as a one-time consultant.

Alice looks less anxious this time. I explain my role as consultant and the boundaries it imposes. I want her to be clear that I will not be her therapist.

"Why did you want to see me again?" I ask, after the formalities are concluded.

Alice responds by repeating some of the things she told us in the first interview: her doubts about Adam, her economic worries, her worry about facing the same problems as her parents. Having little else to go on so far, I put these worries into a hypothesis.

Hypothesis 1: Alice is anxious because her perception of Adam as unlikely to provide financial security confronts her with the risk of a marriage strained by the kind of economic pressures to which her parents' marriage (she thinks) succumbed. She is fearful of a similar fate, with its burden of social failure, and with the added risk that, like her mother, she would have to give up her children. So far this hypothesis merely takes what Alice has told me and restates it in cause-and-effect terms. To see what truth there is to it, I look for confirming material.

"Tell me more about your parents' financial troubles," I ask her. "You were a young girl then. What do you remember about it?"

Alice sighs and proceeds to tell me at some length about the hardships she remembers. Much of it she heard about years later, when she and her brother were reunited with her mother and her second husband. What she says does support the importance she is giving it in facing her current decision. I test the idea further with a question about Adam. "Are you sure Adam is going to be unsuccessful like your father? Does he remind you of him?"

Alice laughs. "No, not at all. They're completely opposite personalities."

"So what makes Adam a failure?"

"He doesn't take money seriously. We'll go out, and he'll spend all his money on things to show me a good time. I don't think he's a practical person."

I offer an alternative idea as a test interpretation.

"Maybe it just means he's in love with you and wants to show it."

"Maybe. Actually he says he's got a lot saved up. He thinks we'll be able to make it without a problem."

So my hypothesis is further strengthened, not only by the confirmatory information about Alice's perception of Adam's money handling, but also because my little test interpretation elicited some new information—namely, that Adam saves his money and has an eye toward the future. Another idea occurs to me. Hypothesis 2: Alice is afraid marriage would interfere with her acting career.

"Alice, one more thing. Are you afraid that getting married would interfere with the acting career you've been working so hard at?"

Alice looks puzzled and shakes her head. "Plenty of successful actors are married," she says. "I don't think that has anything to do with it."

My role as a consultant might appear to give me more leeway to ask these questions that may seem "out of the blue" and to take a more active role than I might want to pursue as a therapist, but my behavior would be no different if I were to be her therapist instead of Arthur. The therapist must function as a consultant at the start of any case. You cannot begin therapy until you know what, if anything, needs to be done, and finding out is the initial, consultation phase of any therapist-patient relationship. At this point, I mention to Alice that we have only about 15 minutes left. Is there anything else she wants to talk to me about?

Alice hesitates and looks embarrassed. She stares at her shoes. Then she sighs again and squares her shoulders. "Yes," she says. "I have to tell somebody about my stepfather."

She goes on to relate that her stepfather sexually molested her on two occasions: once when her mother was at a parents' night at her brother's school and the two of them were alone in the house, and then again when the family had gone swimming in a nearby lake—he had come up to her in the water and grabbed her from behind. That time she turned on him angrily and told him to get away from her or she would call her mother over. Her stepfather backed off, and he had not approached her again.

Should I make a supportive comment here about her having handled the incident well for a young girl? Probably not. I have too little information at this point and would risk a blunder. A supportive comment could strengthen our rapport, but as a consultant I might better avoid stimulating expectations or provoking contrasts between my style and Arthur's. More important, I want to keep the consultation separate from treatment. I have not yet put together a treatment plan and do not know whether my seemingly helpful comment would fit in.

Alice gave these accounts in a flat and apparently unemotional way. She answers my further questions about the incidents in the same detached manner. As the interview ends, I tell her that I am glad she has been able to bring up this difficult issue, that I will talk to Arthur about how the therapy might help her with it and with other problems, and that Arthur will meet with her again. After Alice leaves, I ask Arthur how he might formulate the case.

"We have a 28-year-old single woman," he begins, "with a chief complaint of pervasive anxiety. She works as a sales clerk but wants to be an actress. She's worried about getting married, probably because her parents' marriage was bad and ended in divorce. She meets criteria for generalized anxiety disorder. We might also consider an adjustment disorder, except it's gone on too long for that."

Arthur has given a competent but limited and essentially static formulation. Other than weakly linking Alice's ambivalence about marriage to her parents' history, his formulation is a summary of two hours of interview material into a few sentences that focus on making a supportable diagnosis. His diagnostic conclusion fits the facts but by itself provides little guidance about how to treat the patient. There are a variety of possible treatments for generalized anxiety disorder, including the use of medication, which she has already rejected. Arthur's formulation does not help us decide which one might be the best. To see how we might develop a more useful formulation, we must go back to the assessment and assemble the evidence we collected.

In answer to our *three questions*, we learned that Alice chose the clinic because her family doctor recommended a mental health referral when she declined to take a pill for her nervousness, and the clinic was all she could afford; that she came at this point in time to forestall a decision about marriage; and that she wants treatment to take away her anxiety and help her decide whether to marry her boyfriend. From the history, we learned about her parents' troubles. She told us she was "given up" to an aunt for two years when she was 11 and that after she rejoined her mother and new stepfather, he sexually molested her on at least two occasions. She kept the abuse a secret, and despite revealing it in the interview, she seems to have walled off her feelings about it. It seems likely these events, too, are contributing to her difficulty with the idea of getting married.

We can augment Arthur's summary with this additional material and arrive at a more complete formulation: We have an unmarried woman getting close to 30, hoping for a career on the stage, whose life seems stalled and unfulfilling. She has yet to come to terms with her early bad experiences with her parents and later sexual abuse by her stepfather. She lives with a diffuse but persistent apprehension, worsening over the last year, that interferes with her work and brings on headaches and irritability. The increased anxiety coincides with her deepening relationship with her boyfriend and especially with his interest in marrying her. These developments have confronted her with more intimacy and commitment than she may feel ready to take on. The formulation could be further improved by noting that the caretaking adults in her life have mostly let her down. Her parents could not sustain their marriage, and her father left her. Her mother gave her up to an aunt. Her stepfather violated the parent-child boundary by his sexual interest in her. She considers her aunt the only good caretaker, and she lost her as well. The result seems to be a general distrust of relationships, like that with Adam, that contain a promise to take care of her.

The formulation now takes note of particular problems that might be translated into treatment objectives. Should the treatment focus on her anxiety symptoms, her floundering stage career, her unresolved feelings about her parents, her traumatization by her abusive stepfather, her fears of intimacy, or her conflicted relationship with her boyfriend? Should it try to deal with all of these or only one of them? Should it take them at random or recognize an order of priority? To answer these questions is to plan a course of treatment.

REFERENCES

Bateman AW: Integrative therapy from an analytic perspective, in Integration in Psychotherapy: Models and Methods. Edited by Holmes J, Bateman AW. New York, Oxford University Press, 2002, pp 11–25

Bremner JD, Steinberg M, Southwick SM, et al: Use of the Structured Clinical Interview for DSM-IV Dissociative Symptoms in posttraumatic stress disorder. Am J Psychiatry 150:1011–1014, 1993

Eells TD (ed): Handbook of Psychotherapy Case Formulation. New York, Guilford, 1997

Endicott NA, Endicott J: "Improvement" in untreated psychiatric patients. Arch Gen Psychiatry 9:575–585, 1963

Frances A, Clarkin J, Perry S: Differential Therapeutics in Psychiatry: The Art and Science of Treatment Selection. New York, Brunner/Mazel, 1984

Frank A, Eisenthal S, Lazare A: Are there social class differences in patients' treatment conceptions? myths and facts. Arch Gen Psychiatry 35:61–69, 1978

Goldstein AP: Patient expectancies and non-specific therapy as a basis for (un)spontaneous remission. J Clin Psychol 16:399–403, 1960

Greenson R: The Technique and Practice of Psychoanalysis, Vol 1. New York, International Universities Press, 1967

Guaron EF, Dickinson JK: Diagnostic decision making in psychiatry, 1: information usage. Arch Gen Psychiatry 14:225–232, 1966

Gunderson JG, Phillips KA, Triebwasser J, et al: The diagnostic interview for depressive personality. Am J Psychiatry 151:1300–1304, 1994

Horowitz MJ: Formulation as a Basis for Planning Psychotherapy. Washington, DC, American Psychiatric Press, 1997

Luborsky L, Auerbach AH: The therapeutic relationship in psychodynamic psychotherapy: the research evidence and its meaning in practice, in Psychiatry Update: American Psychiatric Association Annual Review, Vol 4. Edited by Hales RE, Frances AJ. Washington DC, American Psychiatric Press, 1985, pp 550–561

Malan DH, Heath ES, Bocal HA, et al: Psychodynamic changes in untreated neurotic patients. 2. Apparently genuine improvements. Arch Gen Psychiatry 32:110–126, 1975

Meissner WW: The Therapeutic Alliance. New Haven, CT, Yale University Press, 1996

Narrow WE, Regier DA, Rae DS, et al: Use of services by persons with mental and addictive disorders: findings from the National Institutes of Mental Health Epidemiologic Catchment Area Program. Arch Gen Psychiatry 50:95–107, 1993

Perry S, Cooper AM, Michels R: The psychodynamic formulation: its purpose, structure, and clinical application. Am J Psychiatry 144:543–550, 1987

Regier DA, Narrow WE, Rae DS, et al: The de facto US mental and addictive disorders services system: Epidemiologic Catchment Area prospective 1-year prevalence rates of disorders and services. Arch Gen Psychiatry 50:85–94, 1993

Regier DA, Kaelber CT, Roper MT, et al: The ICD-10 clinical field trial for mental and behavioral disorders: results in Canada and the United States. Am J Psychiatry 151:1340–1350, 1994

Robins LN, Wing J, Wittchen HV, et al: The Composite International Diagnostic Interview. Arch Gen Psychiatry 45:1069–1077, 1988

Sandifer MG, Hordern A, Green LM: The psychiatric interview: the impact of the first three minutes. Am J Psychiatry 126:968–973, 1970

Sperry L, Gudeman JE, Blackwell B, et al: Psychiatric Case Formulation. Washington DC, American Psychiatric Press, 1992

Williams JBW, Spitzer RL, Gibbon M: International reliability of a diagnostic intake procedure for panic disorder. Am J Psychiatry 149:560–562, 1992

Winston A, Pinsker H, McCullough L: A review of supportive psychotherapy. Hosp Community Psychiatry 37:1107–1114, 1986

Zarin DA, Earls F: Diagnostic decision-making in psychiatry. Am J Psychiatry 150:197–206, 1993

Chapter 8

FROM
FORMULATION TO
TREATMENT PLAN

Arriving at the final treatment plan is a two-stage process. The first stage takes place within the mind of the therapist, as he or she translates the formulation into a working blueprint for the therapy to come. The second stage is a transaction between therapist and patient in which the therapist's ideas are presented to the patient, reviewed, revised, and advanced toward a consensus. In this second stage, therapist and patient must reach an agreement about what they will try to accomplish and how they will do it.

EARLY PLANNING STAGE:
CONSTRUCTING THE PLAN

The therapist may begin to assemble the plan elements during the initial interview, the planning process running in the background, so to speak, as the assessment occupies the foreground of attention, but a period of quiet reflection may be needed as well. Experienced therapists might take a few minutes of silent review during the interview, telling the patient they need to think about what they have heard before making a recommendation. For the therapist less practiced in treatment planning, or for the experienced planner confronted with a complex case, it is useful to reserve some time after the assessment and present the treatment plan in a subsequent session.

In any case, the starting point, as always, should be a decision as to the AIM of the therapy. Who determines the AIM will vary. Sometimes the therapist will be in a better position to synthesize the patient's hopes and expectations into a coherent objective. The therapist seeks to answer the question, "If my work with this person can bring about the best possible outcome, what would that be?" The key word is *possible*. Many desirable outcomes may occur to the therapist, but only one will represent what this particular patient, with his or her unique combination of time, money, energy, intelligence, motivation, and personal strengths and liabilities, will be capable of attaining. We are not looking for the ideal outcome, only the best outcome. Sometimes the patient will come in with a clear and reasonable interest in achieving a given result. Remember the most important of our three questions: What does the patient want? If what the patient wants is realistic and can be achieved with the therapist's skills and the patient's abilities, it can be the designated AIM, even though the request might require further investigation and discussion.

The decision about the AIM may be reached at any point in the assessment process, subject to revision if significant or critical material emerges later, but often the AIM that seems right early on will still look like the right answer as more information develops. The advantage to an early decision about the AIM lies in its being the organizing principle for all of the planning that follows.

Let us briefly review the way finding the AIM is an exercise in inductive reasoning. The assessment provides the relevant history, clinical observations, and diagnostic possibilities from which emerges a group of problems. They may be independent and constitute a simple list, or they may be interconnected, a kind of problem matrix. The therapist must pull these materials together into a single abstract concept that embodies the desired outcome of the therapy.

Once we have the AIM in mind, we can ask a series of questions that progressively define our plan. The question that follows from the AIM is "If this is what we want to achieve, what must happen for us to get there?" The answer provides the GOALS that our patient must reach. Knowing the GOALS, we can ask, "What kind of treatment approach will work best with this patient?" The answer for each GOAL is the STRATEGY we will use. The choice of TACTICS for each treatment modality follows from a similar question: What therapeutic techniques will make this therapy successful?

Contrast this top-down, inductive approach with its opposite. If we collect all the data about the patient, we can then attempt to deduce from it what elements are most likely to lead to a beneficial outcome. Suppose, for example, that in our assessment of Ernest the Edgy Engineer[1] we listen to his story of escalating worry over a minor engineering error, his episode of sexual impotence, the deepening depression that followed, and his leave of absence from work. If we group the historical facts together with the impressions from our interview with him, we can identify problem areas and their possible relationships. We can deduce, in other words, that the two episodes Ernest considered failures brought on his low mood and that all three factors precipitated the leave of absence that confirmed his own low opinion of himself. At this point, we have a formulation, but we do not yet have a plan. Deduction alone does not provide us with one. Deduction tells us that leaving his job brought on these serious problems, but it does not tell us what to do to solve them.

Which one of Ernest's problems is the most important? Should we concentrate on one of them? On two? Can we expect to ameliorate them all? How would we accomplish this result? What kind of therapy will best help him overcome these problems? A list or matrix of problems leaves us without a logical approach to answer these questions. True, we could take them one at a time and apply our best efforts to each, or we could take our best approach and plug him into it with the hope that solutions will emerge. Suppose, for instance, that we specialize in cognitive group therapy. We could invite Ernest to join the group and see what progress he can make. But whether we choose the one-at-a-time approach or simply pick the most credible treatment for the entire problem list, we have not used the formulation to plan treatment.

By contrast, the inductive approach helped us to recognize a coherent overall plan for Ernest. We considered three ideas that were reached inductively—that is, we answered the question, "What kinds of treatment outcomes would address this list of problems?" We selected one of the ideas—the AIM to return him to his prior level of function—by eliminating the other two: We judged characterological reconstruction to be beyond his abilities and resources, and we eliminated getting him quickly back to work without a significant change in his outlook because it was too risky. Applying inductive logic supplied us with the ideas, and our clinical judgment provided the means to choose among them. Armed with a single organizing idea, we could then select the particular objectives—the GOALS—of our work with the patient. Working top down from the AIM, we selected those GOALS whose achievement could bring that AIM to fruition. Working top down from the GOALS, we selected the

---

[1] See case vignette, Chapter 2, pages 19–20.

best STRATEGIES to reach those GOALS and then the TACTICS to carry them out.

Clinical Example: Alice the Anxious Actress

As a further illustration of turning the formulation into a treatment plan, we can continue with the case of Alice.[2] Our formulation identified half a dozen clinical issues: her presenting symptom of anxiety, her slow progress as an actress, her conflicted memories of her mother, her abandonment after her parents' divorce, her stepfather's sexual abuse, and her ambivalence toward her boyfriend's offers of intimacy and marriage. We must decide whether to deal with some or all of these issues, which ones should take priority, and in what order.

Consider the following formulation.

We know from the interviews that her most immediate reason for seeking treatment was Alice's uncertainty about the marriage proposal. We surmised, in fact, that she might have sought therapy as a temporizing move, a way to put off the decision. Her anxiety symptoms, which were long-standing although somewhat worse over the last stressful year, were her "admission ticket," the acceptable reason for asking for help. When asked what she hoped for from the therapy, Alice answered: less anxiety and help with making her decision about her marriage proposal.

A first marriage is an important transitional step. The couple leaves their families of origin, to whom they still have strong emotional ties, and join together to form their own, new family, the family of procreation. Alice hesitates on the threshold of this transition. Our formulation is that her biological parents provided her with a poor example to follow, a model of tension, fighting, and ultimately divorce. Her stepfather shattered her trust when he crossed the parental boundaries to approach her sexually. Adam's marriage proposal raised economic concerns and stimulated misgivings about whether he was reliable and trustworthy. Her long-standing and pervasive anxiety had a corrosive effect on her confidence in her ability to make the right choice. We can also link what Alice told us about her mother and stepfather to the dilemma she feels about Adam. When her mother gave her up to her aunt after the divorce and when her stepfather molested her, Alice was left with unresolved pain and grief, with uncertainties about whom to trust, and with apprehension about the future. These experiences affected her relationship with

---

[2]See case vignette, Chapter 7, pages 97–101.

Adam, an impact that came to a head when he proposed to her, and they contributed to her indecision about marriage.

Using this formulation, we can now begin the treatment plan, starting at the top.

The decision whether to marry Adam could be selected as the AIM for Alice, not only because Alice has identified it as the issue for which she wants treatment but also because so much of her past history and present experience tie into it. We can tentatively state the AIM as *help Alice decide whether to marry Adam,* but we must include more factors. From her history, we know Alice can make this judgment more readily if the effect of her traumatic family experiences is neutralized. At present, these experiences contaminate her judgment and fuel the ambivalence she feels. We might also assume that her generalized anxiety, whatever its source, limits her ability to reach a decision about marriage. She is anxious when she is with Adam, and she feels less able to rely on herself. Her anxious mood supports her belief that she cannot make a choice or if she does that she is not "well enough" to handle the presumed stresses of the relationship. Finally, she seems to have some real uncertainty about Adam himself, but given her earlier experiences, it is likely that her view of Adam is distorted. The real Adam and the Adam onto whom she may have projected her own fears and doubts combine to produce an ambiguous figure that makes her judgment more difficult.

If we include all these considerations in our construction of the AIM, we must modify our statement of it. We would hope she can make a decision about Adam on his merits, with as little influence as possible from the effects of her early experiences with abandonment and abuse. We want her decision to be free of irrelevant conflicts, of ideas that may have seemed true in her childhood but that are no longer real and present dangers. We want her to avoid, to use a term not currently in fashion, a neurotic choice. Our amended AIM would be to help Alice make a realistic, conflict-free decision about marriage in general and Adam in particular.

Our effort to turn the ideas in the formulation into a plan of treatment not only has led to a statement of the AIM but also has suggested the GOALS Alice would need to reach if that AIM were to be realized. These GOALS would include enough integration of her early traumatic family experiences to keep them from contaminating her current relationship with Adam, a reduction in her level of anxiety to the point where it interfered minimally with her decision about marriage, and resolution of the ambiguities about Adam. Let us take these GOALS one at a time.

Goal 1: Integrate Early Traumatic Family Experience

Alice's childhood was unusually stressful. Parental divorce and early sexual abuse are unfortunately all too common in our society, but having to live with relatives after the divorce is less so. Alice had to cope with all three of these stressors during the first half of her life, and the cumulative effect shows in the present. It is perhaps tempting to think a successful period of therapy could reverse these bad effects and make her whole again. This hope may be realistic, or it may represent a "rescue fantasy" on the part of the therapist. We would need to know more about Alice and to examine our own feelings about her before we could decide, but the more important considerations are that Alice's expectations are more limited and that she does not ask for this transformation. We might convince her otherwise, but at this stage we need not try. The AIM we have selected does not justify such an ambitious undertaking, and to pursue it might require so extensive a period of therapy that Alice's opportunity to examine her marriage choice could slip away from her. We might reconsider this extended work later on, if Alice wanted to do so, but for now, her needs are better served if we address the childhood traumas only to the degree that they bear on her relationship with Adam.

Goal 2: Reduce Generalized Anxiety

Again we must consider a good-enough result rather than a perfect result. The AIM we chose for therapy does not require that she be free from every trace of excessive anxiety, only that it is reduced enough so that it does not interfere unreasonably with her decision about Adam.

Goal 3: Reduce Ambiguity About Adam

Alice's need to decide about Adam's proposal of marriage suggests that he should be the focus of at least some of the therapy time and energy. It is not enough to consider the way her childhood shaped her general outlook about intimacy and marriage; we must also address the way those experiences may have distorted her perceptions of him. We want her decision about marrying him, whether it is yes or no, to be based on the real Adam.

Now that we have the AIM and the GOALS in our plan, we can consider which STRATEGIES we might use to reach them. As usual, we must judge Alice's ability to work within the available modalities—where she falls, in other words, on the expressive-supportive continuum—and then select the best STRATEGIES for the particular GOALS of this therapy. Alice

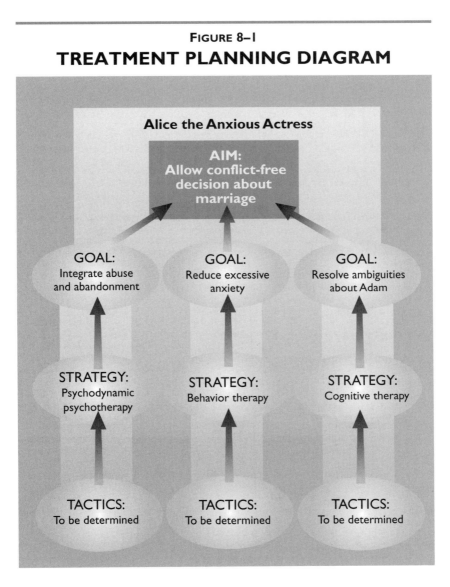

FIGURE 8–1

TREATMENT PLANNING DIAGRAM

Alice the Anxious Actress

AIM:
Allow conflict-free decision about marriage

GOAL:
Integrate abuse and abandonment

GOAL:
Reduce excessive anxiety

GOAL:
Resolve ambiguities about Adam

STRATEGY:
Psychodynamic psychotherapy

STRATEGY:
Behavior therapy

STRATEGY:
Cognitive therapy

TACTICS:
To be determined

TACTICS:
To be determined

TACTICS:
To be determined

shows no major deficit or mental illness, and she seems intelligent and motivated. Her verbal and social skills are adequate. All in all, she seems to belong closer to the expressive than to the supportive end of the spectrum. We can therefore select appropriate therapeutic modalities across a fairly wide range.

We might choose a psychodynamic approach for the first GOAL: integrating the earlier traumas into Alice's adult outlook. She was a helpless young girl when these things happened to her, but she now has independence, experience, and mature resources. The defensive operations she used at those earlier ages, as well as the experiences themselves, are frozen in time, locked in her frightening memories and seen in the present as though through the eyes of a child. To the extent she can reexamine those issues, she may finally come to terms with them and be able to move forward in her life. Because she is apparently unwilling to accept medication for her anxiety state, a behavioral approach would make sense for the second GOAL. For the third GOAL (resolving the ambiguities about Adam), we might consider a cognitive approach as the STRATEGY.

I might choose one group of STRATEGIES, someone else a second mix, and a third therapist might select an entirely different set. The particular STRATEGY employed should be appropriate and potentially effective, but therapists can make use of the modalities with which they are most comfortable, competent, and experienced. Our planning is illustrated in Figure 8–1. If I were treating Alice, this diagram (my handwritten version of it) would be in my case notes.

LATE PLANNING STAGE: NEGOTIATING THE AGREEMENT

So far, therapist and patient are likely to have had an unequal relationship. The therapist has been active, set the agenda, and controlled the interview. The patient has been a relatively passive participant who presented a complaint, told his or her story, and submitted to the therapist's examination. They have now reached a critical step in the planning process that requires a more equal and cooperative collaboration. If the treatment plan is to succeed, patient and therapist must agree on it.

As a practical matter, it is often useful to initiate the discussion of a treatment plan by telling the patient what you think and how it all fits together—in other words, to share your formulation with your patient. How much to reveal and in what terms are matters of clinical judgment, but in my experience, patients are relieved and encouraged by hearing that their story makes sense to you and that you have some ideas about what has happened to them. The therapist can make this presentation in a somewhat formal manner, one that signals the end of the assessment period and the beginning of joint planning, saying, for example, "Well, I've listened to everything you've told me, and now I want to take a few moments to tell you how it looks to me and why your problems have reached this point." You might then proceed to summarize the main issues and say something about the reasons for them. The patient may have questions or additional information to add, but after a reasonable discussion of the formulation, it is now time to invite the patient to join with you in planning the treatment to come.

Patient and therapist have a mutual interest in planning the treatment, and they share joint responsibility for its success. This idea has been recognized in the relatively sparse literature on treatment planning. It is captured in the term *negotiated consensus*, introduced by Levinson et al. (1967). Lazare et al. (1975) characterized the patients' role in the transaction as "customers" who approach therapists with one or more "requests," both open and covert, and who have the option of taking their business elsewhere if dissatisfied with the services offered. Their summary advises:

> In seeking and weighing the merits of various treatment alternatives, therapists need to be encouraged to begin where the patient is at. By this we mean that the therapists should elicit and respond to what kinds of help a patient wants and thinks he needs. By encouraging the patient to voice his treatment preferences, the therapist not only promotes the patient's sense of autonomy and self-esteem, but cements the formation of a therapeutic alliance, and learns what treatment the patients will be most likely to accept…and will benefit from. (p. 68)

Lazare (1979) later outlined the issues and the procedures of the negotiating process.

Seeking a consensus was well summarized by Nurcombe and Gallagher (1986). They presented it as a process that begins with the therapist showing respect and caring for the patient while demonstrating his or her expertise. Next, the therapist must address conflicted areas. Patient and therapist may differ over the problem to be addressed, the results they will seek, the methods to be used, the conditions of treatment, and the nature of their relationship. Conflict may be explicit or implicit, direct or displaced, conscious or unconscious. Reviewing general negotiating principles, Nurcombe and Gallagher suggested developing a consensus about the nature of the problem, clarifying the issues by organizing them in a useful way, establishing priorities, and educating the patient. Specific negotiating techniques included making a concession, providing a sample treatment, sharing control with the patient, confronting and clarifying areas of significant resistance, and using another therapist as a consultant. If these efforts founder and the negotiation stalls, they advised postponing the negotiation, offering a compromise or a unilateral concession, and if all else fails, threatening to end the relationship.

Whatever the reasons, on either side, failure to reach a therapeutic agreement will almost certainly threaten to derail the therapy somewhere down the line. It then requires a much greater effort to keep it on the tracks, and sometimes the result is a train wreck.

Reaching Consensus

The more successfully therapist and patient reach an overt, satisfactory agreement about their work together, the more likely it is that their work will have a good outcome. It is not enough that the therapist make a full assessment, formulate the case, and construct a comprehensive treatment plan. Unless patients participate in refining the plan, see their own views and needs reflected in it, and agree to collaborate with the therapist in fulfilling it, the treatment will struggle and may ultimately fail. An open discussion of the issues favors reaching such an agreement. Therapists must know what patients want and respect their reasonable requests. As experts, therapists bring to the discussion their knowledge and experience, and they can educate patients about what is or is not possible. Patients bring their knowledge of themselves, what they want from the therapy, and their ideas about how this should happen. The procedures used to reach agreement are less important than the commitment to do so.

It is not unusual, however, for both sides to keep what they know to themselves. Therapists and patients can be extraordinarily reluctant to make the initial effort at reaching a consensus: "It is as if there were a conspiracy between both parties in which the patient agrees not to say what he wants and the clinician agrees not to ask" (Lazare et al. 1975, p. 557). Patients may fear rejection or dismissal of their requests. They may not recognize their responsibility for sharing the planning. The same difficulties that brought them to the therapist—emotional distress, problems with relationships, troublesome personality traits—may block their participation in the process. Therapists may believe they know what the patient wants without having to ask, but experience shows this belief is likely to be misleading. They may assume that the patients' "real" requests are unconscious wishes. This assumption overlooks the legitimate expectations patients bring to the interview, even if unconscious factors help to form them. They may worry that the patients' requests will overwhelm their ability to help or will undermine their professional status.

This variety of motives and expectations can influence what each will reveal to the other. Therapists may feel no need to justify their expert status by explaining what they want to do and why, assuming the patient is knowledgeable and does not need their information. Patients may be intimidated by the therapist's expert status, reluctant to reveal their expectations for fear of looking foolish or of insulting the therapist, or they may hold the therapist in awe and believe they lack the right to state their views and preferences. Both therapists and patients may have other reasons as well.

Therapists are in the better position to guide the process toward a consensus. They know the importance of reaching one and have the expertise to facilitate it. Through their assessment and formulation, therapists evolve plans that can be shared with the patient, tested against the reality of the patient's responses, and modified if they do not match. They may have to persuade the patient that the plan will be in the patient's best interest.

Ideally, to reach consensus, each side will fully express its views of the critical issues: what the problem is, what the outcome of therapy should be, what steps they must take to get there, and how they will take those steps. They must agree, in other words, not only on the problem but also on the AIM, GOALS, and STRATEGIES of the therapy. Through discussion, modification of their views, making concessions, and adapting their ideas to those of the other, they can arrive at a point where their positions are almost congruent and the differences that remain are inconsequential. A full expression of views often requires a good deal of therapeutic effort to overcome distortions from unconscious motives, consciously concealed apprehensions, distractions from the main task, and the substitution of less important issues. This work can occupy more than a little therapy time, but it is time well spent. The more solid the consensus at the beginning, the better the chances for success as therapy proceeds.

Clinical Example: Alice the Anxious Actress

To illustrate the negotiation process, let us imagine that my work with Alice did not end with the consultation but that I am continuing as her therapist. I would begin with a statement to Alice about what I thought her story added up to. I would, in other words, offer her my formulation, edited of any jargon and presented in terms that invited further discussion.

"Now that we've had a chance to go over what's been happening to you," I might say, "why don't I tell you how it looks to me? And I'd like you to tell me where you think I might be off the mark or where something doesn't make sense to you." I am telling Alice not only that I have an "expert" opinion to give her, but that I also expect her to participate as an active partner and correct me when she thinks I am wrong. This stance tries to empower Alice right at the start to be a mutual participant in our work.

"You've told me a little about the really rough times you went through as a kid. First your parents split up, then you lived as a kind of foster child with your aunt, and even though she was good to you, I'm sure it was hard to be away from your mother. And then you finally got back with her, and her new husband treated you terribly by making sexual advances."

Alice's eyes are moist. She says, "It wasn't their fault. They did the best they could."

As I asked her to, Alice has given me her own viewpoint about her family. She excuses them with a clichéd phrase. If she were already in therapy with me, I could respond to her defense of her parents by doing one of the following:

- Challenging the denial: "Even your stepfather? Was he doing his best?"
- Exploring the affect behind her tear-filled eyes: "You look like you're ready to cry."
- Acknowledging the pain: "This is really hard for you, even when I'm the one saying it."
- Offering an interpretation: "I wonder if you're trying to excuse them because otherwise it's too painful to think about."

At this stage, I usually would not want to offer any of these comments. They are all tactical interventions and would mean I have started psychotherapy before Alice has even agreed that we should do so, much less what she would accept in the way of treatment conditions, and a response from her might lead to further exploration that would divert us from the treatment plan.

However, there are two reasons why I might want to make one of these interventions despite the above caveat. The first would be if I felt Alice needed a "sample" of the therapy to see whether it was one she could accept. The sample could be as brief as a single intervention or long enough to consume more of the session. It could even be a longer trial period after which we would agree to step back and decide whether to continue that approach. This step would almost always occur, if at all, farther along in the treatment planning process. My discussion with Alice is at such an early stage that an offer of a sample treatment now would be premature.

The second exception would be to make a "test intervention." If I were uncertain whether to use a particular approach, I might try out one of the TACTICS associated with it to see how my patient responded. I might, for example, offer Alice the interpretation about excusing her parents to protect herself from painful feelings. Her response would help me assess whether she was capable of confronting those feelings, and I would also hope to see how defensively she might respond to an interpretation, even one as "on the surface" as this one. She might close down with a denial or a perfunctory but false agreement, or, the more encouraging predictor, she might open up an area of new material. Either response would tell me more about her ability to work within an introspective approach. Although these exceptions would actually be in the interests of advancing the treatment planning process, I choose to go on with my explanation to her.

"They may have done their best," I say, "but it still seems to me that those years shaped your outlook about other people in general and about the idea of marriage. I think your past experiences might intrude into your relationship with Adam and add to your uncertainty about whether to marry him."

Now, by explaining what I see as a cause-and-effect relationship between her childhood and her present uncertainty about her possible marriage partner, I am, of course, making a kind of interpretation, but it summarizes a part of the overall "case history" and stays within the task of reaching consensus.

"I don't know," Alice says. "When I worry about getting married, it's because I worry about Adam. I don't even think about those bad times from before."

"All right," I say. "The most important thing you've told me is that you don't know which way to decide about marrying Adam. You don't know whether to accept him or put him off some more and maybe lose him."

"Oh, you're right about that. It's like my mind is paralyzed."

"Yes. And when I asked you what you wanted from therapy, you said you wanted to be able to make a good decision about him. I agree with that, and that's what I think the therapy should do for you. We'll know the therapy has succeeded when you feel you can make a decision about getting married that you feel good about."

So I have stated the AIM, as I formulated it. I carefully said that her decision does not have to be the perfect decision or even the right one. She will know that only with time, and I do not anticipate she will wait around in therapy for that time to pass.

"That sounds good," Alice says after thinking a moment, "but how in the world are we going to do that?"

"I have some thoughts about that, but before we get into them, I want you to consider my idea and tell me whether you fully agree with it. Is that what we want the therapy to do, to help you make a clear decision about getting married? If there are other things you want or you don't agree with me, let's talk them over before we go on."

"No, I do. That is what I want. But part of the problem is that I'm so nervous. I've never been what you'd call a calm person, but the way I am lately is terrible. I can hardly keep my mind on what I'm supposed to do."

"Yes, you told me about that. And I think being so nervous is a problem, too. In fact, I think it gets in the way of your relationship with Adam, and it would help you decide whether to marry him if you weren't so terribly anxious about everything, including him."

Alice nods.

"So now I've told you two things I think are paralyzing your decision, even though you're not sure about the first one. I think the stresses in your family and the big increase in your anxiety level explain a good deal of the problem."

"Well, I didn't mean I didn't go through some bad times with my family. I just said I try not to think about them."

"And maybe that's the problem. Not thinking about them keeps you from putting those bad experiences behind you. You can't think about them because they make you feel bad all over again, and they do that because it probably feels like you're still in them. We want them to be bad memories of the past, not battles you have to keep fighting over and over again."

"And how do we do that?"

"We have to talk about them here, a little at time, as much as you can handle. When you were a little girl, you couldn't act on your own. You didn't have the experience and the independence you have now. If we talk about what happened, you can look at those past experiences as the grown-up woman you are now."

In this imaginary dialogue, Alice and I have now discussed the AIM and two of the three GOALS in my treatment plan. We would still need to discuss the third GOAL, of examining her perceptions about Adam to see which are valid and which may be distorted. To the extent her perceptions are distorted by her past experiences with her family, the two GOALS would overlap. That is not a problem in doing the therapy, but for clarity in setting GOALS for the treatment plan, it is helpful to treat them as entirely separate.

Finally, we would have to discuss to some extent what type of therapy I would propose for each of the three GOALS: the STRATEGY level of the planning hierarchy. As I mentioned above, a cognitive-behavioral approach could justifiably be used for all three GOALS, but I have chosen separate STRATEGIES in this illustration. I would describe a little about psychodynamic psychotherapy and explain why I thought it could help look at the way past family experiences might influence her now. I would also describe the need for a cognitive approach to sort through her feelings and attitudes toward Adam to give her a clear picture of him and therefore a more rational choice. Again we would review my proposals and discuss them in whatever depth was required to arrive at a consensus.

Alice previously rejected medication for her anxiety. Perhaps I could convince her otherwise, but behavior therapy offers a reasonable and effective alternative. I might suggest using the behavioral approach for a period of time and, if the anxiety had not responded, reconsidering the medication.

I have said relatively little to Alice about the tactical level of the plan. It is difficult at this early stage to have a clear idea about what techniques will work best. Even if I did, my explanations would probably be more effective once we are actually engaged in the work. The process of educating the patient goes on throughout the course of the therapy regardless of the particular treatment modality employed. The more patients understand about the work we are doing, the more cooperative and engaged they are likely to be.

DISCUSSION

Agreement about all four levels of the plan is not equally important. The most important element is the AIM. Unless therapist and patient agree on that issue, the rest of the plan will be irrelevant. We must come to a consensus with the patient about what we are trying to accomplish. If the patient sees the problem as one thing and the therapist sees it as something different, and if what the patient wants differs from what the therapist is prepared to work on, they will operate at cross-purposes, and the result will almost certainly be a treatment impasse.

The next most important element is agreement on the GOALS. Therapists must formulate their cases to identify the specific objectives that will contribute to the overall outcome both parties seek. The patient must understand the proposed GOALS and agree with them, but patients may have GOALS of their own. Sometimes these are expectations and hopes that either do not contribute toward the AIM or represent some unrelated and less important outcome, one that might be the basis of another piece of therapeutic work but that is not helpful with the present effort. If the patient's GOALS, however, contribute more effectively to the outcome than the ideas of the therapist, they should be adopted.

Agreement about STRATEGIES is less important still. First, the patient may not have the knowledge to evaluate whether a STRATEGY is the best one for the task envisioned and must, more than ever, rely on the therapist's expert knowledge. Yet the patient may have valid objections to a proposed STRATEGY. Perhaps it is one that was tried by a previous therapist with little benefit. Perhaps it is a value judgment, such as Alice's reluctance to use medication for her anxiety symptoms. There might be cultural or social beliefs that affect the choice. Even though more knowledgeable, the therapist must reach agreement with the patient to expect reasonable compliance.

I have already mentioned that tactical considerations are the least important area of agreement, but they are not exempt. Patients still need to understand and accept what is being asked of them before they can participate successfully. This requirement holds true even in the case of paradoxical techniques, where a straightforward explanation risks destroying the intended effect. Haley (1963) advocated such a paradoxical technique: The therapist typically instructs the patient to undertake an unpleasant or burdensome task. Confronted with such an ordeal, the patient is encouraged to "give up" the symptom. An example of this approach was the suggestion to a patient with insomnia that he stay awake and out of bed each night to polish his hardwood floors, ostensibly so that he would be too busy to worry about not sleeping. The patient disobeyed by returning to a normal sleep pattern. The insomnia sufferer had to understand the cover story about keeping busy and agree to follow the therapist's instructions even though he found them distasteful.

So far, I have described the negotiating process as though it involved only rational, objective considerations about the merit of which both parties could agree or disagree. In practice, distortions and various behind-the-scenes forces are present even at the beginning of the therapy relationship and threaten to interfere with the working alliance. Fortunately, these influences are mitigated by three factors.

The first is that planning discussions usually occur at the beginning of therapy. At this very early point, the potentially disruptive forces tend to be quiescent. Transference issues, cognitive distortions about the therapist, and the like have not yet been fueled by the therapeutic process. To the extent they arrive with the patient, of course, they are a factor to be reckoned with, but except for psychotic patients or those with severe character disorders, the immediate emergence of disruptive distortions is unusual.

The second mitigating factor is that planning the therapy lends itself to a dispassionate discussion. Although the plan is about the patient and reveals some things about the therapist, the topics themselves are relatively neutral. After all, we are not talking so much about the patient's personal history and presenting problems as we are about the possible approaches to deal with those topics. This distancing tends to move the discussion away from the emotional aspects of the patient's life. Although the issues may be loaded with feelings and conflict, the planning process itself is a less emotional exercise.

The third factor involves the concept of the "real" relationship between patient and therapist. It exists separately from the therapeutic relationship, and patients usually understand that they and the therapist are both interested in succeeding. We rely on the patient to recognize the objective and rational elements that underlie and support the therapy effort.

That having been said, the negotiating process is still vulnerable to fear, suspicion, displaced anger, and other disruptive influences the patient might bring into the consulting office with the first visit. To the extent they interfere with the attempt to reach a consensus, these distorting influences must be identified and dealt with like any others until they diminish sufficiently to go on with the planning effort. That process might take a good deal of time, but it is not time wasted. In fact, the effort to discuss, debate, educate, disagree, offer alternatives, make concessions, and reach compromises—the whole negotiating process—can identify and ameliorate some of the interpersonal and dynamic issues that brought the patient into therapy in the first place. It can therefore be a positive therapeutic process. With some patients, the negotiating process can extend throughout the therapy. When treating patients with personality disorders, the resolution of this process may *be* the therapy.

REFERENCES

Haley J: Strategies of Psychotherapy. New York, Grune & Stratton, 1963

Lazare A (ed): Outpatient Psychiatry: Diagnosis and Treatment. Baltimore, MD, Williams & Wilkins, 1979

Lazare A, Eisenthal S, Wasserman L: The customer approach to patienthood: attending to patient requests in a walk-in clinic. Arch Gen Psychiatry 32:553–558, 1975

Levinson D, Merrifield J, Berg K: Becoming a patient. Arch Gen Psychiatry 17:385–406, 1967

Nurcombe B, Gallagher RM: The Clinical Process in Psychiatry. Cambridge, UK, Cambridge University Press, 1986

Chapter 9

PUTTING IT ALL TOGETHER

In the preceding chapters, we have looked at the individual elements of a treatment plan and the separate steps needed to reach a therapeutic contract. Of necessity, this approach presented a somewhat fragmented picture of what should be a continuous and seamless process. We can now follow a single case from its beginning to the completion of its contract.

CASE STUDY: FREDDY THE FRIGHTENED FRESHMAN

The setting is the student mental health service of a New England college, a few days before the brief Thanksgiving vacation. My initial interview with Freddy, a 19-year-old freshman, was arranged by the intake nurse. After screening him, she decided he was not at risk and set up a routine appointment. Her referral sheet says only, "Freshman with academic stress." I introduce myself to Freddy in the clinic waiting room and invite him into the office. His handshake is firm but he looks ill at ease, and his voice is shaky.

"So," I say, "what can I do for you?"
"Well, the day I called here, I found out my grades from the midterms, and they were a lot lower than I expected. C's and D's mostly. I got a B minus in History of Art. So I went to see my adviser, Mrs. Frank."
"Was she helpful?"

"She asked what the problem was. I said I didn't know. I study all the time, but when I think I've learned it, nothing stays with me. When I got into the exams, my mind went blank. It was an awful feeling."

"You're not used to that."

"No. In high school I was one of the best students. I was in honors classes for everything. I just don't understand why this is happening to me." Freddy looks pained and embarrassed. "I told Mrs. Frank I didn't realize how hard college courses would be. I never had to write these long papers. And they don't always tell you what to study. You're supposed to do a lot of work on your own, in addition to what they tell you to read. Well, I was telling all this to Mrs. Frank, and all of a sudden I started crying. It was embarrassing. I didn't even know it was going to happen. And Mrs. Frank looked like she was as surprised as me." He stops and stares at the floor.

"What happened then?"

"She said I needed professional help. She gave me the number here and said I should call for an appointment. She said lots of people get help here."

"That's true. We do see a lot of people. What kind of help do you think you need?"

Freddy hesitates. "I don't think I'm crazy or anything. I need help learning how to study at a college level, so I can get my grades up. I study as hard as I can, and that's all I do. I don't go out; I don't go to any of the social events here. I just study."

"Are you nervous about studying?"

"I'm nervous all the time. I don't have any friends here. I met a few guys down at meals, but after we leave the dining room, I don't see them. I don't think they're interested in me. I had a lot of friends in high school, but here, I haven't been able to make any."

"Because you spend all your time studying?"

"That, and because I'm scared. I'm scared I'm going to fail and have to leave here." His voice becomes husky and I can see his eyes are moist. "And everybody's counting on me."

"Who's everybody?"

"Everybody back home. My parents. Friends. They're expecting big things of me. If they knew how it really was..." He lets the sentence hang.

"You don't talk to them about it?"

"Oh, yeah, I do. I call home about every other day, in fact. I kind of tell them about it, not as bad as it really is. Only that I'm having a hard time getting going."

"And what do they tell you?"

"They're very supportive, really. They tell me not to worry so much, that I'll start to catch on pretty soon. They tell me to take it easy and not worry about the grades."

"But you're not convinced."

"I feel better after talking to them, my mom especially. But I can tell they're worried too, no matter what they say to me. I can feel there's a lot of tension there. About me. They get this funny way of talking, like they don't want me to know they're really worried."

"Who's at home?" I ask. "Tell me a little about the family."

"I have a great family. My father's a lawyer, pretty successful and all. I really admire him. I want to go to law school after this. In fact, my sister is graduating this year from the law school here. She's on the law review, did really well. My brother is doing well, too. He's a junior at another school. Right now he's in Germany in a college exchange program. Junior year abroad."

"How about your mother?"

"I'm really close to her, being the baby of the family like I am. My grandmother, too. She lives with us. She keeps saying she hopes to live long enough to dance at my wedding."

"Your family's very impressive. Do you feel they're a lot to live up to?"

"Yes, I do. I'm afraid I won't be able to do as good. I'm going to be the one to let down the family name."

"That sounds like something a father might say."

"Yeah, you've got it. He doesn't say it about me. He just says we all have to be proud of our family name and live up to it."

As the interview goes on, Freddy tells me more about his family and his success in high school. His wistful tone prompts me to say, "You sound like you have a touch of homesickness."

"I guess a little. But I don't run home. I stay here every weekend. I'm even going to be here over Thanksgiving. Studying."

"So you won't see the family until the Christmas break."

"Yeah." He looks at the floor, dejectedly; then he shrugs and straightens up. "I'd like to go home for Thanksgiving, but staying here is the right thing to do."

He tells me about his two roommates. He thinks they handle their work much better and are often out of the room at campus activities. Freddy stays behind trying to catch up on assignments. Occasionally, he goes to the library to work there. His only social time is at meals. I also learn that anxious ruminations interfere with his efficient use of study time. Too often he simply stares at his work without seeing it and worries about himself. His anxiety stays with him at other times, making him uneasy when he talks to other students or faculty and further inhibiting him from social and academic contacts. It turns out he has been seeing Mrs. Frank at least once a week, mostly "just to talk." He describes her as a nice older woman, "a little like my mom."

ASSESSMENT

By this point, we have used more than half the interview time. I want to reach some understanding with Freddy before he leaves today about what, if anything, he and I should do about his situation. I have an initial impression about this young man's problem. Certainly he is not terribly ill. I see no evidence of major depression, incipient psychosis, or any long-standing disorder. His mental status seems benign: He is alert, cooperative, pleasant, with mildly pressured speech and an anxious but euthymic mood. He shows no psychotic phenomena or, in answer to my direct question, suicidal ideation. His judgment seems a little immature but nevertheless intact. For the record, I might put down a diagnosis from DSM-IV-TR (American Psychiatric Association 2000) of adjustment disorder with anxiety. The previous diagnostic manual had a more specific subtype: adjustment disorder with academic inhibition (DSM-III-R) (American Psychiatric Association 1987), but he meets criteria for both. Neither label tells me how best to help him.

Does he need psychotherapy? The college provides remedial courses and even individual tutors for students who need extra academic help, and I can point him toward these resources. My concern is that he will not get enough help of the kind he needs from those sources alone. I can reassure him ("It's normal to have some problems adjusting to college in your first term") and send him back to his adviser. Mrs. Frank may have felt out of her depth when Freddy started to cry. She may have interpreted crying in a male student as indicating a serious emotional problem, but freshman advisers do not casually send students to the mental health service. They often sense when there is real trouble, and her judgment merits attention. I suspect Freddy's problem is more than merely low grades. His concerns—about his family, for example—go beyond adjustment to a new school. He is consumed with worry about his family's reaction. His anxiety interferes with his concentration and suggests a level of tension greater than expected from the stress of freshman year. At this point, I lean toward providing some therapy for him rather than normalizing and reassuring him.

I have listened to Freddy for answers to the three assessment questions: Why here? Why now? What does he want? I have also listened for clues to the AIM, the best outcome. I have also assembled a formulation from the history and from my impressions of Freddy as the interview progressed. As it happens, Freddy has, directly or indirectly, supplied answers to my three assessment questions. The answer to the first question (Why here?) is that Mrs. Frank, his adviser, told him he needed "professional help" and directed him to the student mental health service. Her referral raises a question about his motivation for therapy. Because it was not his own idea, he may be less open to a psychotherapy approach than to the academic help he wanted from her. The answer to the second question (Why now?) is also clear. The precipitant was his shock at his poor showing on the midterm exams.

Might Freddy have found his way to the mental health service without this catalyst? Possibly. He had been feeling lonely and isolated during these first two months away from home. After his high school successes, he had a sense that his folks back home were expecting big things of him. He felt he was floundering and would let everyone down. Yet he had not sought help before the midterm grades were posted, and if he had done a little better he might have muddled along through the rest of the school year. He might well have improved on his own, given more time and opportunity. That the referral came about, at least indirectly, through the sudden increase in his level of anxiety tells me that even if he starts therapy, he might not stay with it when things settle down again. I can also expect that for him to want to stay in therapy, he will likely have to see it as providing real help with his academic problems. Finally, his reaction to the sudden precipitant on top of two months of anxious struggle suggests that his defenses were stretched thin before the exams and he had relatively little in reserve.

Freddy has a clear answer to the third question: He wants to improve his study habits. This is not a request for mental health services, because Freddy thinks of his problem as more academic than emotional. Although I expect that lowering his anxiety level would help him study more effectively, I cannot redefine his current distress entirely as a mental health problem. I will need to acknowledge his specific request and let him know I appreciate the issue that is important to him. At the same time, I have supporting evidence for the hypothesis that the stress of leaving home plays an important part in his troubles as well. He will be more likely to embrace a treatment plan that responds to his realistic request, but I will have to educate him about why I think he needs to work on more than his academic problem. I suspect Freddy has an inkling of the wider problem already. He readily accepted his adviser's mental health service referral, and here he is at the interview. He should be willing to listen to ideas that help him both with studying and with his feelings of distress about being away at school.

The answers to my three assessment questions suggest that Freddy's referral to the mental health service by his academic adviser was appropriate. His crisis involves more than an academic issue. His midterm grades were a relatively minor academic setback; after all, he did not fail anything. Yet the result looms over him as incipient failure, and he hopes, perhaps unrealistically, to avert future academic trouble with better study habits. These conclusions help me frame the problem more clearly.

FORMULATION

My initial formulation is as follows: This 19-year-old single male college student presents with an eight-week history of anxious mood, difficulty studying, and social isolation. He was referred by his academic adviser after he cried in her office. The precipitant was getting back his lower-than-expected midterm exam grades. He comes from an intact, successful family with high expectations. He is somewhat homesick. He perceives his adviser as a motherly woman and sees her frequently. His outstanding high school achievements suggest that his problems here result from his emotional state rather than a lack of academic and social skills.

The interview raises several questions whose answers would help shape my formulation. Is he fearful of challenging his father or his successful older siblings? Is his poor academic performance a covert attempt to return to his mother and grandmother within the nurturing family? Is overstudying a means of avoiding the anxiety of new peer relationships? I might raise other questions from a more "cognitive" reference point: Has *all* of his study effort been a failure? Do his fellow students truly have *no* interest in him? Does his family *really* believe he is letting them down?

To conceptualize the optimum outcome of my work with Freddy, however, I must complete the formulation. I want one that recognizes all of the above elements but generates ideas that point me toward the AIM of the therapy. The most important issue for this young man is his struggle with a transition toward adult independence. When he left home, he left the security and approbation of his family. At college, he faces a trial of early adult independence, but within this protected environment he feels insecure and alone. He is more than merely homesick; he is stalled in an important phase of his life. This developmental difficulty expresses itself in Freddy's overconcern with the family's approval, his anxiety about meeting their standards, and his delay in connecting himself with people and activities in his new "college family." He seems overly attached to Mrs. Frank, perhaps as a substitute for his distant mother. Not only is his academic "failure" on the midterms is the result of his anxiety and its interference with effective learning but it also keeps Freddy more tied to the family through his worried telephone calls, through his preoccupation with what they are thinking about him, and through his childlike helplessness and dependence. No wonder he surprised Mrs. Frank by bursting into tears like a young child.

The historical data from my single interview is sparse, but the core issue can be restated as this hypothesis: Although physically separate from his family, Freddy remains emotionally tied to them, too much in the role of a dependent child and unable to develop further toward adult independence.

PLANNING

My formulation now suggests the AIM of my work with Freddy. If the problem is developmental, it follows that the AIM ought to be mastery of the transitional task. The challenge Freddy faces is to complete a normal transition: to establish his early adult independence. If he can resume his progress toward young adulthood, therapy will have a successful outcome. This clear statement of the end point does not mean our work together will be either easy or short; clarity of purpose does not guarantee either. Nor will it be necessary to keep him in treatment until he fully achieves adult independence. That might be quite a long while and would risk substituting a dependence on me for the relinquished dependence on his family. Therapy can end when he is moving toward independence and appears capable of completing the transition on his own. The AIM here is his resumption of the developmental process, not his completion of it.

My next step is to decide what GOALS, if met, will allow Freddy to realize this AIM. What prevents this young man from progressing in his development? From the history, we know that he is continuing to cling to his family, that he is neglecting to establish new peer relationships, and that he is failing to apply the study skills from his successful high school days to the new challenges of his college work. These inferences lead us logically to three GOALS: 1) develop more emotional independence from his family, 2) establish new peer relationships, and 3) study more successfully. If Freddy can achieve all three, the likely result will be progress in his adult development.

What is the difference between the AIM and the first GOAL? The transition to adulthood includes more than emotional independence. It includes the ability to be physically separate without discomfort, financial independence, the freedom to consider forming a new family through marriage and procreation, and above all a modification of personal identity. The therapy does not contemplate seeking these changes. He is already physically away from home. Financial independence will obviously have to wait, as will almost certainly a new family, until he is finished with school. Although his adult identity may evolve during therapy, it is too broad a GOAL for the time and resources available through the student health service at the college. The AIM here is simply to get him started toward adulthood, and the GOAL of more emotional independence from the family can be a catalyst to help him move forward.

The importance of the second GOAL is that new peer relationships will provide a substitute for the weakening of his family ties. If we expect him to let go of the family, he will need his peers as at least temporary emotional ties. Some of these college friends may be much more than that.

The first two GOALS, then, connect more closely with the AIM: If he achieves more emotional distance from the family while strengthening his relationships with peers, he will have moved from a more childlike position toward that of a young adult.

The third GOAL is important because it is the specific request he brings to the initial interview. I want to meet this request if I can. It will strengthen his interest in the therapy. More success as a student promises to bolster his self-confidence and to provide an important source of gratification.

In contrast to the three GOALS I plan to discuss with Freddy, let us consider three inappropriate GOALS.

1. *Provide emotional support until he is stabilized:* An offer of supportive help would rest on the assumption that given time to work things out for himself, Freddy will use his current abilities and psychological defenses to solve his own problems. It is possible he would do so, but this very limited GOAL presupposes a different and more limited AIM, something like "resolution of the crisis," and fails to acknowledge the developmental issue that lies behind it. Freddy might very well do better on his next set of exams, given some remedial help and emotional support, but then again he may not. If he is really stuck at a developmental impasse, supportive work will fall short of what he needs.

2. *Provide symptomatic relief:* Freddy is mildly anxious and somewhat discouraged, although not clinically depressed. Perhaps some anxiolytic medication would help him concentrate better on his work and approach social interactions more successfully. This GOAL—reducing anxiety—again rests on the assumption that crisis resolution is the desired outcome of his therapy. Freddy has not asked for medication, and his attitude in the interview leads me to believe he may be reluctant to accept it. Giving him medication with these marginal indications could have negative effects. It might suggest to him that he is really "ill" or seriously disabled, undermining his shaky self-confidence and increasing his tendency to cling to the nurturing family. The effects of the drug on memory and alertness might impair his learning and make him feel even more different from his peers than he does already. For these reasons, symptomatic relief through medication is not a helpful GOAL for Freddy.

3. *Undertake a reconstructive character analysis:* This more ambitious GOAL would require a quite different formulation than the one I proposed; namely, that Freddy struggled through a significant earlier conflict that now manifests itself as fixed and maladaptive personality traits. His self-defeating reluctance to compete with the more successful members of his family, for instance, might represent such a fixed pattern. Perhaps he needs to work through his oedipal fear that it is too dangerous to challenge his father. Maybe his overdependency on his mother and grandmother reveals his failure to resolve even earlier issues.

On a second look, though, these concerns probably overstate the degree of Freddy's difficulty. The assessment provides insufficient evidence to support this more ominous formulation, and he does not demonstrate a level of impairment sufficient to justify undertaking such a major therapeutic task. The practical issue of a time constraint would also argue against this GOAL, because he will be at the school for only 28 weeks out of the year. For Freddy, this GOAL is neither justifiable nor realistic.

The GOALS I have selected—to enhance Freddy's emotional independence from the family while strengthening both his relationships with college friends and his use of study skills—more closely match my formulation that he needs some limited help in proceeding toward adult independence.

A process of discussion, education and negotiation must take place before Freddy and I can proceed. I will include him in as much of the planning process as he can manage, and I hope he will agree with the plan I am constructing, but Freddy's wishes and ideas may persuade me to modify the plan until we both feel it is the right one.

As a brief illustration of how I would record this interview and my initial plan, see Figure 9–1.

My three GOALS are only abstract ideas, and I still need concrete methods for achieving them. Treatment planning must now move to the next level: defining the STRATEGIES by which Freddy and I could work together. STRATEGY selection is a more technical decision than planning GOALS, and I must use my professional expertise and judgment. Even here, however, I may tell Freddy what approaches I am considering for our work together, and I will discuss the reasons for my choices if he wants to hear them. His acceptance of my methodology is part of our therapeutic contract.

An effective therapist is often comfortable and competent with more than one therapeutic modality. Not every problem is best handled

FIGURE 9–1

TREATMENT PLANNING DIAGRAM

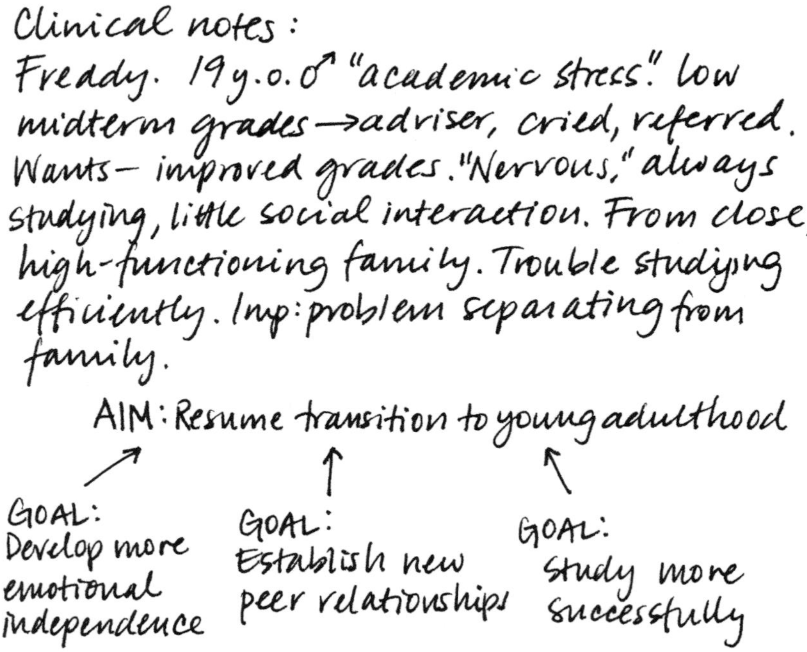

Clinical notes :
Freddy. 19 y.o. ♂ "academic stress." Low
midterm grades →adviser, cried, referred.
Wants— improved grades."Nervous," always
studying, little social interaction. From close,
high-functioning family. Trouble studying
efficiently. Imp: problem separating from
family.

AIM: Resume transition to young adulthood

GOAL:
Develop more
emotional
independence

GOAL:
Establish new
peer relationships

GOAL:
Study more
successfully

through a cognitive-behavioral approach, nor can a psychodynamic psychotherapy provide the best answer to every clinical challenge. Selecting the most appropriate STRATEGY is part of the therapist's art. In thinking about how to help Freddy accomplish the GOALS we are setting, I decide to use three different therapeutic approaches:

1. For "emotional independence," a psychodynamic approach, perhaps focused on the dependency issues that are close to the surface.
2. For "new peer relationships," a cognitive approach that examines his negative overgeneralizations about his efforts to make new friends. (This approach might also be helpful in examining his ideas about his ability to study and about his family.)
3. For "study more successfully," I have two STRATEGIES in mind. Each uses a behavioral approach: a) identify the skills he already possesses and develop structured tasks to emphasize them, and b) help him develop new study skills as needed.

Note that I have been more specific about these STRATEGIES than I was in earlier discussions. I have selected not only a particular therapeutic modality (psychodynamic psychotherapy, cognitive therapy), but I have also indicated what I wanted each one to focus on (dependency issues, making new friends). This further planning step is, in effect, notes I have made to myself. The more detailed the therapist makes the plan, the more useful it will be in conducting the therapy.

Selecting the TACTICS needed to carry out these STRATEGIES is the most familiar part of the planning process.

1. Exploring the dependency dynamics includes the four basic steps in psychodynamic psychotherapy: *identify* dependency issues, *clarify* their meaning in Freddy's life, *interpret* the dynamic issues involved, and allow him to *work through* them until fully integrated.
2. Correcting negative overgeneralizations involves a cognitive approach to identify negative overgeneralizations and ideas, to contrast them with more realistic assessments, and to reexamine their true importance. In other words, false ideas would be challenged and tested.
3. Helping Freddy study more effectively can be done through two STRATEGIES. Each requires its own TACTICS: a) "enhancing existing study skills" through behavioral interventions using direct advice and perhaps "homework" or structured tasks between visits, and b) "developing new study skills" by collaborative use of the school's remedial programs. I could refer Freddy to another helpful person within the college system—the writing tutor, for instance—for direct academic assistance, and support the tutor's work in our therapy sessions through my continued interest. One kind of help does not preclude the other.

Unhelpful TACTICS might include direct or confrontive oedipal interpretations. An adult might be able to deal with these ideas, especially in an anxiety-provoking brief therapy, but they might be too much for Freddy, still an adolescent. They could prove more frightening and drive him back toward the shelter of the family. A passive, completely nondirective (Rogerian) approach—simply restating whatever Freddy said in an effort to help him clarify his own thinking—could also be problematic. Freddy is still somewhat childlike and would be more likely to respond to a more direct approach. We must respect his interest in getting help with the practical problem of ineffective studying.

Another experienced clinician might well select other STRATEGIES and TACTICS or use those above in pursuit of different GOALS. For example, if a cognitive-behavioral STRATEGY were used to pursue all three

GOALS, the TACTICS might include suggestions to decrease telephone calls to the family, to attend campus activities likely to attract desired peers, and to use the college's study resources, such as the writing tutor. They could work as well or better than my preferences. The important thing is to make deliberate and thoughtful choices about how to carry out the planned work.

Our TACTICAL decisions conclude the planning process, and Figure 9–2 shows how my notes in the clinic chart might look at this point. My treatment plan includes Freddy's original request—to improve his study habits to get better grades—and thus "begins where the patient is at," but it expands his request to deal with the issues behind the academic problem and redefines the therapy as an attempt to energize his struggle with a stalled developmental task. I would use this written planning diagram in later sessions and refer to it in my clinical notes, noting which goals we worked on and what progress or problems occurred.

NEGOTIATING THE AGREEMENT

Now that I have a plan, my next step is to discuss it with Freddy. We are nearing the end of the initial interview, and I would like to reach an agreement with him before we stop. We need to decide, first of all, if we are to proceed any further. This might be our only meeting. Freddy can decline my offer of psychotherapy or decide he does not want to work with me. He might feel better enough as a result of this one interview not to want further help. When I interrupted my report of the interview, you may recall, Freddy was telling me he saw Mrs. Frank, who reminded him a little of his mother, every week, "just to talk."

> "Is that enough help?" I ask. "I mean, considering how anxious and lonely you've been feeling, do you think that talking with a trained therapist might be more helpful?"
> "Would I have to stop seeing Mrs. Frank?"
> "Not necessarily. She's still your freshman adviser. But it sounds to me like she might have felt she was going a little outside her adviser role when you showed her how strongly these problems were affecting you."
> "You mean when I cried?"
> "That, and probably the things you had talked to her about before that. Did you tell her about how you worried you'd let the family down?"
> "Yes. She told me I shouldn't worry about that. She was sure I'd get with the program."
> "Did that help?"
> "I felt better for a little while. Then the worries took over again."

FIGURE 9–2

TREATMENT PLANNING DIAGRAM

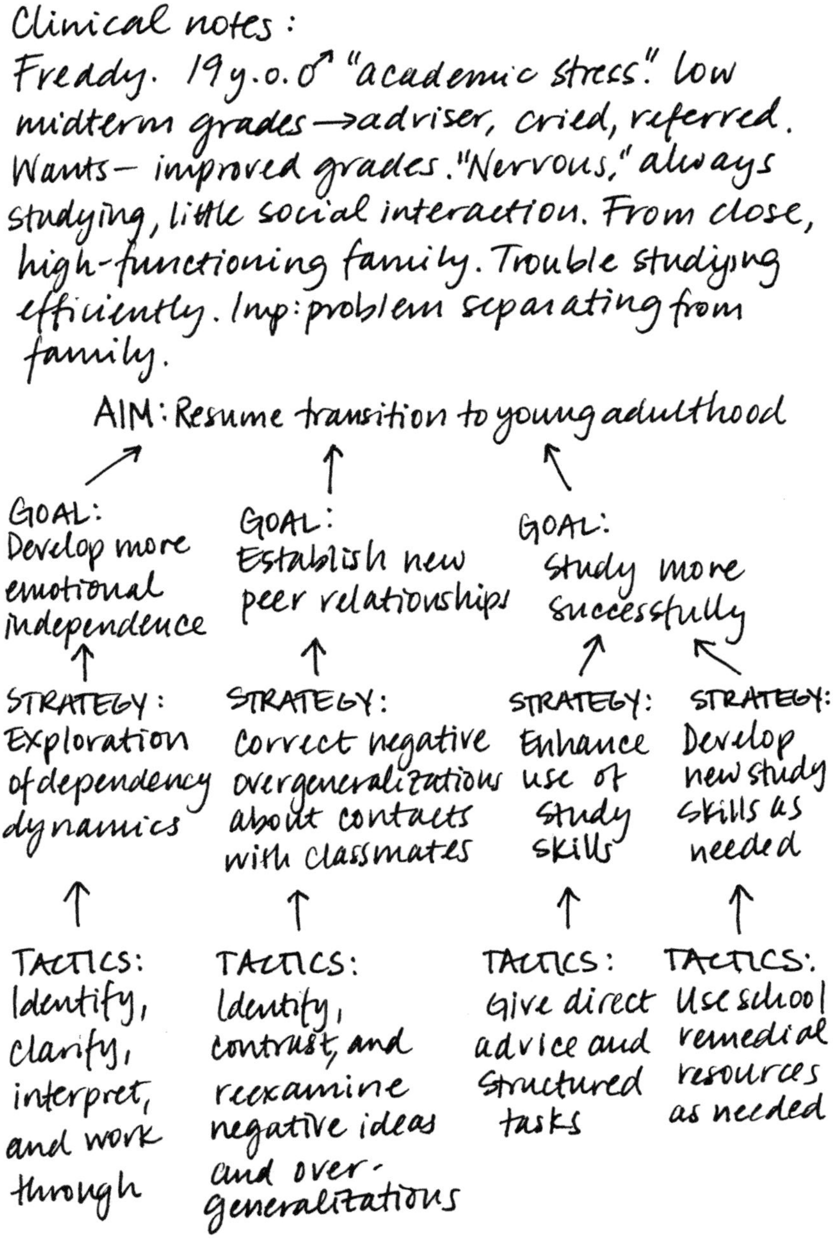

Clinical notes:

Freddy. 19 y.o. ♂ "academic stress." Low midterm grades→adviser, cried, referred. Wants— improved grades. "Nervous," always studying, little social interaction. From close, high-functioning family. Trouble studying efficiently. Imp: problem separating from family.

AIM: Resume transition to young adulthood

GOAL:
Develop more emotional independence

GOAL:
Establish new peer relationships

GOAL:
Study more successfully

STRATEGY:
Exploration of dependency dynamics

STRATEGY:
Correct negative overgeneralizations about contacts with classmates

STRATEGY:
Enhance use of study skills

STRATEGY:
Develop new study skills as needed

TACTICS:
Identify, clarify, interpret, and work through

TACTICS:
Identify, contrast, and reexamine negative ideas and over-generalizations

TACTICS:
Give direct advice and Structured tasks

TACTICS:
Use school remedial resources as needed

"Well, that's what I mean. Perhaps it would help to work on those worries here, and you could concentrate on the academic stuff with Mrs. Frank."

"If I came here, would I be seeing you?"

"Yes, if you want to."

"I like talking to you. I guess I could do that."

So far, the negotiation has resolved Mrs. Frank's role (she'll remain as an academic resource), Freddy has agreed to psychotherapy, and I have agreed to be the therapist. I next want to tell him my impressions as a basis for further negotiation. In other words, I will offer him my formulation.

"Let me tell you what I think so far," I begin. "The main problem is that you're having trouble adjusting to college. You described your family as a wonderful group of talented and caring people, and I think it's hard for you to be away from them and to be more on your own than you were back in high school."

"I've been away before. At summer camp. I did okay then."

"Don't you think, though, that college is different? More of a serious challenge? You've already been here longer than a summer camp season."

"Yes, that's true. Being here makes me feel more disconnected from them. And summer camp was playing all summer. I didn't think college was going to be so hard, so much work."

"Maybe it feels like you're moving on with your life now and starting to leave the family. That's a tough step for most people. The funny thing is, the better your family is, the harder it is to move away from them."

"Sure, that makes sense. If they were bad people, I'd want to get away."

"Well, that's what I see as the problem. You've been going along fine all through high school, growing up and learning how to handle yourself. The fact that you did do well up to now tells us you have a good chance of getting over this hurdle and moving ahead with your life."

"I suppose so." Freddy looks anxious.

"I don't mean you need to cut yourself off from the family and pretend they don't exist. You wouldn't want to do that. They're important to you. All I mean by moving ahead is that you can *start* to become more independent. It takes a while for young people to get ready to do that. Finding yourself all alone here at the college was more of a change than you expected. You stopped looking ahead. You haven't been able to rely on yourself. Our job would be to see if we could get it started again."

I have managed to state my idea of the AIM of the therapy in non-threatening terms. Freddy nods and visibly relaxes. We talk some more about what it means to go through a major transition. When I think we are clear on what the therapy should try to do, I introduce the GOALS I have chosen. I start by acknowledging his interest in improving his grades by studying more effectively, and I agree that this result should be an important part of our work together. I tell him that at our next meeting I will have some concrete suggestions about how he could bring about that result. I add that the other problem he is having at school is also very important. He needs to make some new friends and begin to become more a part of college life. Freddy looks anxious again.

> "I don't know if I can spare the time," he says. "I need all the time I have just to keep up with my classes."
>
> "You could be right. I don't know you very well yet. But you tell me you were an honors student in high school, and the admissions committee must have thought you were able to handle the work here. Otherwise they wouldn't have let you in."
>
> "That's true." Freddy smiles for the first time. "Well, I'd like to get to know some people here. I really would."
>
> "Sure. So that's the second thing we should work on. We should take a good close look at your ideas about the people here. You said a little while ago that the guys you met weren't interested in you. Maybe that's not the whole story."

Again, we talk over the idea until I am sure Freddy sees it as a useful GOAL, and then I mention that the third thing we would want to talk about is his family and how he feels being away from them. With this GOAL, he agrees easily enough. It is the topic he has been preoccupied with himself.

We are now at the end of our time. Our initial interview has been productive, especially because Freddy has agreed fairly readily with my suggestions about the treatment plan. There will be more to do next time. I promised him some suggestions about studying better. I will begin some behavioral work to help him enhance the use of his existing study skills, and I will refer him, as necessary, to the remedial resources the school provides. Mrs. Frank could be helpful in doing that. I will also begin to explore with him the generalization "I have to be perfect or no one will like me" as a way of looking at his difficulty with current peer relationships. As Freddy brings up family issues, I will focus on the dependency issues that I suspect lie behind the anxiety about meeting their standards. Reaching an agreement with Freddy has been a smooth process, at least so far. My sense is that he and I have formed a working alliance sufficient to get us started and that the work will have a successful outcome.

REFERENCES

American Psychiatric Association: Diagnostic and Statistical Manual of Mental Disorders, 3rd Edition, Revised. Washington, DC, American Psychiatric Association, 1987

American Psychiatric Association: Diagnostic and Statistical Manual of Mental Disorders, 4th Edition, Text Revision. Washington, DC, American Psychiatric Association, 2000

Chapter 10

THE PRACTICE OF PLANNED THERAPY

After we construct the plan, after we reach agreement with the patient and we start the therapy proper, we begin to implement the treatment plan. How this happens—the actual work of therapy—will vary. Therapists differ in training, style, and experience, and every patient has unique qualities. Just as no two therapist-patient dyads are alike, so no two courses of therapy will run the same. All therapies, however, share three characteristics: 1) progress must be monitored, 2) plans may need to be revised, and 3) therapy must one day end.

MONITORING PROGRESS

To know whether the plan is working, we must review it from time to time. In very active therapies, where things can change rapidly, review might be continuous. In more deliberative therapies, review can be intermittent. From a treatment planning perspective, the purpose of monitoring the plan is to make sure the work continues to be directed at the GOALS with which it began. If we lose sight of those GOALS, the therapy will drift toward standstill.

We need two kinds of measurement for this review. The first, looking for signposts, measures the *process* of therapy. The second, setting benchmarks, measures points of interim *progress.*

Signposts

Every psychotherapy has a characteristic process. A psychoanalyst might recognize a sequence of remembering, repeating, and working through.

147

A group therapist might focus on the development of group cohesiveness and its consequences. A cognitive therapist might observe the gradual dissolution of dysfunctional thinking. Therapists operate with an expectation of some general pattern, often described through specific terminology. We can measure these processes by examining the course of the therapy and looking for their expected patterns. The distinctive phases that mark that pattern act as *signposts* to let us know whether the therapy is on track.

The therapeutic effort can stray off course in two ways. First, the therapist might begin with one approach and then change to another. Someone trained in transactional analysis, for example, might decide a Rogerian approach will better help a patient, start by reflecting the patient's feelings and ideas, but shift later to scrutiny of games and crossed interactions. Second, the patient may agree on a therapy approach at the beginning but find it too worrisome or puzzling to continue. Although some patients will let us know directly that they are having difficulty, others will act out, alter their own part of the process, or simply drop out of treatment. The therapist must recognize the change, either in himself or herself or in the patient, as soon as possible to deal with the problem effectively.

As an example of the use of signposts, suppose we select a behavioral approach to help a male patient overcome an elevator phobia. We decide on two desensitization techniques. In the office, we will ask the patient to close his eyes and imagine himself confronting the open elevator door, then standing in the doorway, then entering the stationary elevator, riding up one floor, and so forth. While this process is under way, we will ask him to undertake the same kind of gradual exposure to a real elevator between his appointments in the office. In this simple example, participation in these two exercises is the pattern of the therapy. Each exercise is a *signpost* of this behavioral therapy plan.

For two weeks, therapy proceeds as planned. At his third appointment, the patient reports he had an upsetting fight with his wife. It made him "so nervous," he says, that he could not face his elevator assignment for the week. He wants to talk about his marital problem instead of to-day's desensitization exercise. The missing signpost alerts us to a disruption of the treatment plan. We have three choices. We can insist he stick to the plan and do the planned exercise. We can explore the marital topic as a resistance to proceeding with the behavioral treatment. We can alter the treatment plan, perhaps by adding "marital harmony" as an additional GOAL of therapy. Whatever we choose to do, we should make a positive decision. If we accommodate the patient's request without making a deliberate choice of one of the three options, we risk losing the treatment plan. If we decide to revise the plan, we must reformulate the case and renegotiate the therapeutic contract. Then we can judge whether we are making the best choice for the patient. The presence or absence of a signpost keeps us alert to whether the treatment plan is working.

The case of Freddy the Frightened Freshman provides another example.[1] For several sessions, Freddy has talked about feeling lonely without his family, and we have implemented our STRATEGY of exploring his dependency feelings. Now he comes in with a big smile and reports he got an A on his latest English paper. He goes on to tell us about his week—amusing things that happened in class, a movie he saw a few nights earlier, what his roommates have been doing. In short, he provides a chronicle of his week. During this narrative, Freddy also mentions that things are going well with the tutor he has been seeing; that he is studying better in the library, where he finds fewer distractions; that he has started studying with another freshman who is in two of his classes and would now consider him a friend. His chronicle contains both "filler information" and elements of other parts of our plan (the GOALS of establishing new peer relationships and of studying more successfully). The missing signpost is the discussion of family relationships. Filling the therapy hour with his weekly activities does not allow time for it, and its absence tells us Freddy is not up to talking about it, at least not today. We must use our clinical judgment to decide whether to mention the avoidance in today's session or wait a week. If we wait and the signpost is again absent, we will have more reason to confront the issue. If we still wait and it does not appear for a third session, the risk of ignoring it is even greater. The longer it is missing, the more likely is its omission significant.

Identifying key parts of the therapeutic process as signposts better allows us to keep track of the progress of our plan. As long as they continue to appear, session after session, we know we are on course with the plan we worked hard to put together. When a signpost disappears, we must consider corrective action.

Benchmarks

Between the initiation of a treatment plan and its completion, we can identify one or more interim accomplishments. These *benchmarks* tell us we have completed at least part of what we hope to do. How long it takes to get there can give us a rough idea of the length of time needed for the

---

[1]See case vignette, Chapter 9, pages 131–133.

rest of the therapy. If we fail to reach a benchmark, or fail to reach it in a reasonable amount of time, then we know our plan is not working.

In the signpost example from Freddy's therapy, we mentioned some of the benchmarks without identifying them as such. One of our GOALS was that he study more successfully. He has started seeing a tutor, shifted more of his study time to the library, and worked with another student on homework assignments. His developing relationship with a study partner is an early benchmark for another GOAL, that he establish new peer relationships.

If we can determine the benchmarks before we start the therapy, or at least early on, we are better prepared to monitor our plan. In the example of the man we are treating for an elevator phobia, for instance, our GOAL may be that he ride to the twelfth floor of his building because that is where his office is located. Our benchmarks might be 1) that he enter the elevator without riding it, 2) that he ride to the fourth floor and walk down, 3) that he also ride the elevator back down, and so forth. For Freddy's GOAL of becoming more independent of his family, a benchmark might be that he calls home no more than once a week and, later, no more than twice a month. Choosing these frequencies does not mean we would instruct Freddy to limit his calls. We might not even tell him about our expectations.

Many times it is difficult to foresee what benchmarks are reasonable until we begin the therapeutic work. We do not know as much about the patient early on as we will later. We learn more detail about his or her life and environment as we continue to meet. This additional information makes it easier to know what interim steps we should look for along the way. Just as we included the planning diagram in our written records, so we should also write down the signposts and benchmarks we have identified. The concrete lists and statements of expected progress make it easier to follow the progress of therapy and to recognize when it is not going as we expected. The written record is also useful in responding to requests for progress reports from third parties and their case managers.

Discussion

As we monitor our patient's progress with signposts and benchmarks, we can be aware when therapy is moving forward, when it is off course, when it is slowing, and when progress has stopped. Without them, these judgments can be difficult, and the only way we might know therapy has stalled is when the patient cancels and declines to make another appointment. If we make a point of being aware of the progress or lack of it each time we meet with the patient, we are more likely to be in a position to identify and correct such problems before they reach crisis proportions.

Monitoring progress is more difficult when therapy is unstructured, when time is unlimited, when the therapy requires a passive therapist, or when treatment GOALS are distant. These conditions might obtain in psychoanalytic or existential psychotherapy, for example. Both are more likely to define the therapist-patient relationship as open-ended, but the effort need not be abandoned even here. An open-ended therapy should begin with an idea about what problems the patient brings and what the therapy hopes to accomplish, including a chosen AIM and the GOALS needed to realize it. Too often in long-term therapies the AIM may be unstated, vague, or never openly discussed and the GOALS may be quite general and poorly delineated, and yet both AIM and GOALS exist, and if the therapist can define them, they may be used to monitor progress.

Therapy can begin with a realistic AIM but become progressively open-ended as GOALS change and blur. Bergin and Lambert (1978), calling this the "deterioration effect," described the significant risks of overdependency on the therapist, unrealistic expectations, and consequent failure, guilt, and self-contempt. These negative effects may produce an interminable treatment, the hallmark of a psychotherapy gone awry.

Amada (1983) described a transitional period during which therapy shifts from a short-term to a long-term modality. This period is characterized by "increasing vagueness" about GOALS that were previously well defined, by diminished activity on the part of the therapist, and by an increase in the importance of transference issues. Unless the therapist takes action, he or she may passively accept the patient's overdependency on the therapy relationship as supportive care or hope that vague long-term benefits will somehow result from an undefined therapy effort. Although psychoanalysis is the most open-ended treatment modality, some of its practitioners are sensitive to this risk. Ticho (1972), as noted in Chapter 4, emphasized the distinction between treatment goals and life goals, the latter being the realization of potentials by the patients themselves, after therapy has endowed them with the tools to make further progress on their own. Gaskill (1980) warned against the "myth of perfectibility" and emphasized the self-analytic function whose attainment by the patient in long-term therapy signals the end of the need for continued analytic work.

The AIM diffusion that undermines a treatment plan occurs when the therapist loses sight of the agreement negotiated with the patient. As multiple treatment objectives replace the single AIM with which therapy started, it becomes progressively more difficult to accomplish them. *Signposts* and *benchmarks* are labels for two rather straightforward ideas. We should watch over the process of therapy to make sure we are doing the kind of work we intend. We should look for and mark the interim accomplishments that tell us we are making progress toward the outcome we want to reach.

REVISING THE PLAN

None of us is perfect, and neither are the plans we make. We start with a limited set of clinical impressions and with an incomplete knowledge of the patient. By the end of our consultation, we hope our skill and experience provide us with a reasonably inclusive assessment that allows us to construct a formulation leading to a useful treatment plan. As therapy proceeds and our relationship with the patient continues, our understanding of the patient broadens. Each additional meeting enlarges the clinical picture with additional history and observations. The new material may strengthen our original ideas, but it may also suggest additional GOALS or more promising STRATEGIES. When the assessment changes, so may the formulation, and a different formulation is likely to require alterations in the treatment plan. Continual reformulation of the case sharpens the focus of the therapy so that the altered treatment plan may contain successive approximations of the truth.

The impetus to reassess the original plan may come from circumstances outside of therapy. The patient may encounter new experiences that can help or hinder the work. New problems may arise, even a major change in life circumstances. Sometimes a third-party payer imposes new limitations or unforeseen conditions. With all of these forces at work, it should not surprise us when treatment plans must be reconsidered. Some may only require fine-tuning, others more substantial modifications, and a few might need to be completely revised. On occasion, the entire plan has to be abandoned and the work of planning must be started over.

To illustrate these various degrees of change, I present four vignettes from the case of Freddy the Frightened Freshman,[2] each illustrating a possible variation, an alternate path therapy might take.

Variation 1: Fine-Tuning a Tactic

In the original plan, I am to give Freddy direct advice with structured tasks to enhance his use of existing study skills. At first this TACTIC goes

---

[2]See case vignette, Chapter 9, pages 131–133.

well. I suggest he spend as much of his study time as possible in the school library, where there are fewer distractions and where the presence of other diligent students might provide some indirect modeling and a supportive work environment. I ask him to keep a log of his library hours and to put in a minimum of four hours a day there. Freddy does this for two weeks and reports he is working better. At the third session, Freddy has forgotten to bring the log with him and is evasive when I ask how the library plan is working. In the fourth session, Freddy tells me he stopped going to the library, he thinks the idea is stupid, and he is studying just as well now in his room. In answer to my questions, he insists nothing happened in the library, or elsewhere, to account for his reluctance to go there. He simply doesn't "like your idea." I identify these changes as a missing signpost. After more investigation, I conclude that Freddy now sees me as a repressive autocrat rather than the knowledgeable authority toward whose suggestions he was previously respectful. In other words, a transference problem has arisen in a behavioral plan. Freddy, the good son, has projected onto me some of his resentment about his family's high expectations of him.

My original treatment plan presented the behavioral STRATEGY as though it would be a simple case of imparting advice, an emotionally neutral transaction. Because it is not (and it rarely is neutral, in therapy or in the classroom), I must fine-tune my plan to include some interpretive work directed at the transference. I might say, for example, "Freddy, you've told me that sometimes your folks seem pretty demanding, that they want to control what you do from far away and make sure you perform the way they think you should. I wonder if you haven't started seeing me the same way. Even though you asked me for advice about how to study better, you also feel I want you to do well for my own reasons." This opening would, I hope, lead to a discussion that reduced Freddy's opposition to my advice. It might also lead us into a productive examination of his family relationships and the difficulty he has in separating emotionally from them. In this example, my formulation has not changed, and I can stay with the original treatment plan, but I have brought in an additional technique as a way to fine-tune my work with him on the GOAL of more successful study habits.

Variation 2: Modifying a Strategy

In the original plan, I proposed to Freddy, and he agreed, that we would talk about his family relationships with the GOAL of helping him develop more emotional independence. As I explore with him some of the family dynamics, I notice a change in his mood. Freddy confirms he is now feeling depressed. At times he thinks he will not be able to stay at school. Today he had the fleeting thought that if he were to be a failure, he would be better off dead. This new material requires a reformulation of Freddy's case. I originally thought Freddy's academic struggle reflected a developmental difficulty in making the transition from dependent child to more independent adult. His emerging depression, however, suggests the focus on dependency issues creates an anaclitic stress powerful enough to affect the stability of his mood. His decision to stay at school over the Thanksgiving break may have contributed to his depressed mood as well. After further assessment, I conclude his mood change is not yet at the level where I need to consider medication, but further probing into the family dynamics may worsen the depression. I must also consider the reality of Freddy's limited availability. He is at school for only about half the year; his stay is interrupted by several school vacations.

My judgment is to continue to see Freddy in psychotherapy and to maintain the GOAL of working toward more emotional independence from his family. I believe it will help if I change the STRATEGY from a psychodynamic approach that might stir up further anxiety about his losing family contact to a cognitive approach that will focus on his dysfunctional ideas about them. He may, for example, believe in the all-or-nothing idea that separating even a little from them means he must give up all contact. I am also influenced in making this strategic shift by the published studies demonstrating the utility of cognitive therapy in helping depressed people. A final point: I am already using a cognitive approach for the GOAL of developing new peer relationships. I will not have to introduce a new STRATEGY but will simply broaden an existing one.

Variation 3: Revising a Goal

In Freddy's original plan, the second GOAL is to establish new peer relationships. Freddy has been isolated and lonely, and he must invest himself in college friendships if he is to distance himself more from his family. He has developed one promising friendship with another freshman, Felix. The two have been doing some of their homework together but so far have not expanded their relationship to include campus social activities. I begin to notice that whenever Felix's name comes up in our discussions, Freddy looks embarrassed, almost guilty, and usually changes the subject. When I ask him about this reaction, he manages to stammer out that he has not told me something. When he was 12, he realized he was probably gay. He knows Felix is (Felix has said so) and he wonders whether he should "try something Felix suggested" to see if he really is what he thinks. This new information about Freddy's sexual orientation requires that we reexamine the issue of *new peer relationships*. Freddy has, in effect, changed part of his original request and introduced a more complex peer relationship problem. These differences compel a change in the therapy GOAL. *Establish new peer relationships* now enlarges to include *and clarify sexual orientation*. Perhaps this complex GOAL is too ambitious. Freddy will still need to make new friends, but he is focused for now on the orientation question alone. I assume, from what Freddy says about his leanings at age 12, that even modifying this GOAL does not fully reflect the underlying issue. That issue will likely turn out to be how Freddy will adapt to his new social role and how he will deal with his family and others about his being gay. At this point, however, the therapy must deal with what Freddy brings to it. He is concerned with the question of whether to test out his feelings with Felix. As we renegotiate the therapeutic agreement, I expect that question to be the only one we can deal with right now.

Revising a GOAL usually requires a fresh look at the STRATEGY and TACTICS that were chosen for the earlier objective. I might, for example, want to broaden the cognitive approach to help Freddy look at some of the assumptions about himself and the issues surrounding gays that could be confusing him. Sometimes it means modifying the AIM of the therapy as well, although in Freddy's case the AIM of supporting his transition to adulthood is still supported by the new GOAL.

Before we go on to the final variation, let us look at the changes we have made in Freddy's treatment plan as they would be reflected on his treatment planning diagram. Although my examples of variations were unrelated—in reality, I would not expect all of them to develop in the first few weeks of treatment—I include all three here for the purpose of illustration. Figure 10–1 shows the revised planning diagram. Note that the TACTICS listed under the STRATEGY to enhance use of existing study skills now include the psychodynamic techniques of dealing with resistance to the behavioral procedure of assigning tasks with direct advice. (Although this combination may seem muddled from a theoretical viewpoint, it is both common and effective in practice.) The second GOAL now addresses the sexual component of peer relationships. Finally, cognitive therapy is the STRATEGY for both the family and peer relationship issues. I would, of course, place this new planning diagram in Freddy's chart.

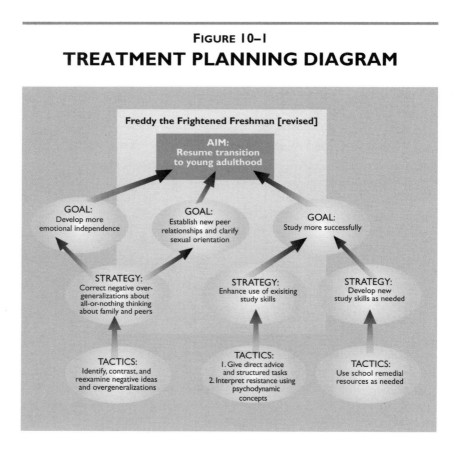

Figure 10–1

TREATMENT PLANNING DIAGRAM

Freddy the Frightened Freshman [revised]

AIM:
Resume transition
to young adulthood

GOAL:
Develop more
emotional independence

GOAL:
Establish new peer
relationships and clarify
sexual orientation

GOAL:
Study more successfully

STRATEGY:
Correct negative over-
generalizations about
all-or-nothing thinking
about family and peers

STRATEGY:
Enhance use of exisiting
study skills

STRATEGY:
Develop new
study skills as needed

TACTICS:
Identify, contrast, and
reexamine negative ideas
and overgeneralizations

TACTICS:
1. Give direct advice
and structured tasks
2. Interpret resistance using
psychodynamic
concepts

TACTICS:
Use school remedial
resources as needed

Variation 4: Setting a New Aim

Freddy's father has a heart attack and is hospitalized. Freddy flies home for the weekend to see him but returns because, he says, his mother wants him to stay in school. He reports that his father appeared comfortable and is expected to make a full recovery. During the next session, Freddy is vague and distracted. He wonders if his family members are telling him everything, if the doctors can be trusted, if his family sent him back to school because something is supposed to happen here. I ask what might happen here. Freddy does not know but says he has had "indications." Such as? There might be a listening device in his room, placed there while he was away. Sometimes he feels like he is being followed. He asks if my office is bugged. He feels something will be expected of him—he cannot tell me what—but he stayed awake all night waiting for a sign.

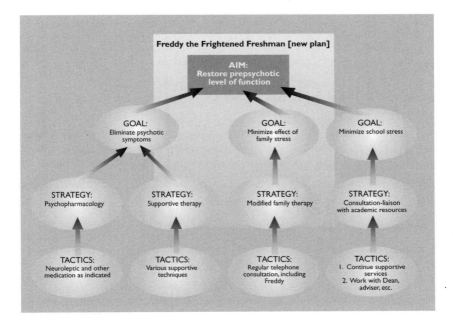

FIGURE 10–2
TREATMENT PLANNING DIAGRAM

Freddy the Frightened Freshman [new plan]

AIM:
Restore prepsychotic
level of function

GOAL:
Eliminate psychotic
symptoms

GOAL:
Minimize effect of
family stress

GOAL:
Minimize school stress

STRATEGY:
Psychopharmacology

STRATEGY:
Supportive therapy

STRATEGY:
Modified family therapy

STRATEGY:
Consultation-liaison
with academic resources

TACTICS:
Neuroleptic and other
medication as indicated

TACTICS:
Various supportive
techniques

TACTICS:
Regular telephone
consultation, including
Freddy

TACTICS:
1. Continue supportive
services
2. Work with Dean,
adviser, etc.

Freddy is developing an acute psychotic disorder. Our treatment plan must be at least suspended, and a new one implemented. Following the same steps as before, I use my new assessment to reformulate the case. The stress of his father's possible death threatens Freddy with a catastrophic loss and with serious consequences even if he survives. His father's potential disability, the disruption to the family, the economic impact, the effect of these changes on his mother—in addition to the potential loss of a loved parent—threaten Freddy's dependence on his family. Psychologically, he feels he is facing abandonment. This stress has precipitated a psychotic attempt to restore his family. Freddy is to be the agent, in some as yet unknown way, of this restoration. Hospitalizing Freddy, either here or at home, remains an option, but at that point treatment passes out of my hands. If I think I can continue to help him and that he can get through this crisis without a hospital admission, I will need a different treatment plan, one based on my new formulation.

The new plan starts with a new AIM: to restore Freddy to his prepsychotic level of function. With its accompanying GOALS, STRATEGIES, and TACTICS, the new plan might look like Figure 10–2. This example illustrates how a significant change in a patient's clinical presentation invalidates a treatment plan and challenges the therapist to address the change with a new approach.

Conclusion

These four variations are examples of circumstances requiring a revision at each of the planning levels. TACTICS may require adjustment to accommodate new technical problems. STRATEGIES may need modification when they no longer help the patient move toward a GOAL. GOALS may need revision as new clinical data emerge that do not fall under the original plan. The AIM may need replacement if the presenting problem changes significantly. In each case, the therapist must make an assessment of the new developments, reformulate the case to take account of the new material, revise the relevant parts of the plans, and negotiate a new treatment contract with the patient.

TERMINATION

Termination has been the subject of much good advice, none perhaps better than from the King of Hearts: "'Begin at the beginning,' the King said, very gravely, 'and go on till you come to the end: then stop'" (Lewis Carroll, *Alice in Wonderland*).

Although few of us would disagree with the King, many find it difficult to decide when they and the patient have come to the end. The original problem, although mostly better, often seems somehow not quite completely solved. New issues have undoubtedly arisen along the way and beg for continued attention. Meanwhile, the relationship between the two participants has become increasingly comfortable and hard to give up. Sending a patient off on his or her own could mean an empty hour. Worse, a new patient will arrive with all the complexity of as yet poorly understood communications, prickly defenses, and challenging transference feelings—not to mention the possibility of an upsetting countertransference as well. Therapy, under these conditions, can continue through inertia or to gratify nontherapeutic ends, becoming static and interminable, or until some change in outside circumstances, such as a geographic change or a loss of health benefits, forces it to end.

Therapists are not always in a position to make the decision about termination. Sometimes patients decide they have had enough therapy, either because they feel they have improved sufficiently or because they recognize the diminishing returns of the later work. They may leave because they conclude they have not benefited. Sometimes outside agents order the therapy to stop. The third-party payer, the "care manager," may conclude the cost outweighs the benefit, or the patient may come up against a prearranged limit on contracted services. These terminations are unsatisfactory, often leaving a residue of frustration, suspicion, or bitterness.

Treatment planning cannot fully solve these difficult problems, but it can bring more clarity to the decision to end treatment. The treatment plan defines termination as the achievement of the AIM. It also specifies what intermediate objectives, the GOALS, will help to reach this end point. When they have attained the GOALS and thus have reached the AIM on which they agreed at the beginning of the work, patient and therapist can agree to stop with a feeling of accomplishment.

Simple as it is to point this out, experienced therapists will immediately find themselves thinking, "Yes, but…" What if the GOALS were not sufficient to bring about the desired outcome? What if the AIM, in other words, requires more to see it achieved? What if the AIM is reached before the GOALS? Somehow, the patient is now where he or she wanted to be yet has not completed the intermediate work. What about those new issues that came up and were not addressed in the original plan? When do they get the attention they deserve? What should the therapist do if the managed-care entity decides arbitrarily that the patient has had enough therapy? We can examine these problems one at a time.

THE RIGHT GOALS AND THE RIGHT AIM

GOALS must be related accurately to the AIM if they are to be productive paths leading to an optimal result. A successful effort requires that unrelated GOALS be rejected or deferred, ambiguous GOALS sharpened, and GOALS that conceal more than one objective clarified or divided into their components. The connection between the GOAL and the AIM must be clear to both therapist and patient. Their agreement on these points is the key to a successful therapeutic contract.

An inappropriate AIM may be the source of the problem. The AIM may be unmeasurable, unrealistic, or even unattainable. Examples of AIMs that therapy is unlikely to provide would include *happiness, self-esteem*, and other vague abstractions. To be useful as an end point, the AIM must be realistic and achievable by the particular patient working in the planned therapy. A poorly constructed treatment plan will inevitably lead to a muddled therapy with an unclear termination point.

Worthwhile but New Issues

Issues unrelated to the original AIM, whether they are recognized at the beginning or emerge along the way, need not be permanently discarded or ignored. Assuming they do not contribute to the current AIM—that is, they are not part of the single most important outcome for the patient right now—they may form the basis for a second course of therapeutic work. In effect, the therapist offers a new opportunity for work at the successful conclusion of the first effort. Patient and therapist reassess the issue, and on the basis of the resulting formulation, they may agree on a new contract. This kind of long-term therapy is a series of shorter therapy periods that continue until all the legitimate AIMs have been accomplished.

Managing Managed Care

A clearly presented treatment plan enhances the dialogue between the therapist and a managed-care reviewer and contributes to a favorable decision. The reviewer may agree with the plan but be required to impose contractual limitations. If so, then patient and therapist unfortunately are faced with one of two choices: either to shrink the treatment plan to fit what is possible under the patient's contract or to agree that the patient will use his or her own resources (if available) to extend the treatment beyond what the third party allows. Although limiting the treatment is less than optimal, a planned decision at least provides a rational response to arbitrary limits and gives the patient as much help as possible under adverse circumstances.

Conclusion

If things go well with the treatment plan, it is easier to recognize the natural point of termination. When the approach of this end point can be predicted more accurately, the working through of the loss involved in termination can begin at the proper point and as an integral part of the process. The sense of satisfaction derived from reaching the planned GOALS and achieving the desired result of the therapy will help to offset the pain both parties feel at the end of a successful and rewarding relationship.

REFERENCES

Amada G: The interlude between short- and long-term therapy. Am J Psychother 37:357–364, 1983

Bergin AE, Lambert MJ: The evaluation of therapeutic outcomes, in Handbook of Psychiatry and Behavior Change, 2nd Edition. Edited by Garfield SL, Bergin AE. New York, Wiley, 1978, pp 139–189

Gaskill HS: The closing phase of the psychoanalytic treatment of adults and the goals of psychoanalysis: "the myth of perfectibility." Int J Psychoanal 61:11–23, 1980

Ticho EA: Termination of psychoanalysis: treatment goals, life goals. Psychoanal Q 41:315–333, 1972

Chapter 11

THE STRUCTURAL IMPASSE

Psychotherapy attempts to help patients realize a significant personal achievement. In planning terms, achieving therapy GOALS moves patients toward the AIM, but as any experienced therapist knows, this process is almost never one of continuous forward progress. The road curves and turns, often forks or doubles back on itself, and sometimes heads off temporarily into blind alleys. The art of psychotherapy lies in the anticipation of these difficulties and the therapist's skill in guiding the therapy along the best available path.

These temporary difficulties result from forces both outside and within the therapy. Outside events may be unrelated, such as a job change that alters the patient's finances, or an overwhelming life event, such as the death of a family member or a patient's sudden serious illness. Within the therapy, relationship issues are a common impediment to progress: a poor match of personalities that gradually becomes a barrier to cooperative work or, more often, transference feelings arising in either participant. Therapists may lack the skills needed for a particular therapeutic endeavor, or patients may have long-standing deficits or fixed limitations that prevent them from profiting from the therapy. These familiar difficulties vary in how easy or difficult they are to recognize. Transference problems, for instance, may arise gradually and become significant roadblocks before they are fully appreciated. Once identified, however, they can be addressed and often resolved in a reasonable way. Therapy arrangements can be revised, relationship issues addressed, and therapeutic approaches modified. An additional, and common, source of difficulty, however, arises from problems with the plan of treatment.

I use the term *structural impasse* to distinguish a difficulty arising from the treatment plan itself, rather than from external impediments or the vicissitudes of a particular therapeutic approach. This structural impasse almost never occurs at the beginning of therapy. Instead, after a productive period in which the therapist may be enthusiastic about a new patient's intriguing problems and the patient may be hopeful the therapy will provide relief and direction, progress slows or even suddenly stops, and there seems to be no way to get the therapy moving again. Although enthusiasm and hope combined to fuel the early progress, the gap between the therapist's agenda and the patient's expectations soon widens, and tension builds until finally it disrupts the therapy.

The unwary therapist may ascribe this tension to more traditional resistance on the patient's part. Attempts at a conventional repair, such as a focus on the transference, may only increase the discomfort. The actual source of the difficulty is that patient and therapist are at cross-purposes, with differing expectations. Unless they realize that the treatment plan is the real source of the impasse, efforts to get the therapy moving are not likely to succeed.

SOURCES OF STRUCTURAL IMPASSE

A structural impasse arises chiefly under three conditions: 1) the plan is incomplete or omitted, 2) the AIM is missing or poorly conceived, or 3) the GOALS are irrelevant, unrealistic, or counterproductive. Problems with STRATEGIES and TACTICS create difficulties with the process of therapy but not with its structure.

Absence of a Treatment Plan

Therapy that begins without a completed plan is likely to end in impasse and may fail altogether. Neither therapist nor patient knows for what purpose they are meeting, why they are talking, or how it is supposed to help. They may each *think* they know the answer to these questions, but their ideas are likely to be completely different. As their perceptions diverge and as tension accumulates, the patient can become frustrated or frightened and drop out of treatment. If the patient remains, both therapist and patient continue to feel increasingly dissatisfied, and to relieve the discomfort, they may allow the therapy to develop into a personal relationship. Unplanned therapy is more likely to persist when it gratifies the nontherapeutic needs of one or both parties. This risk is especially high with patients who feel chronically helpless, excessively needy, or overly dependent and with therapists who are relatively unaware of their countertransference vulnerabilities. The impasse will occur more quickly when therapist and patient seemingly have a mutual understanding but are really in covert disagreement about what should be accomplished. A more subtle variation of this problem is an agreement on a partial plan, one that is not yet finished. When the planning has been hasty and incomplete, its initial progress is likely to slide to a halt. These incomplete or false agreements are more likely to arise if the patient feels less empowered in the relationship and inclined to outwardly agree with what the therapist proposes yet has significant remaining reservations, or if the patient does not fully understand what is being proposed.

A common example of an incomplete agreement is an agreement on process but not on outcome. In my terms, they may agree on the STRATEGY but not on the GOALS or the AIM. A therapist may suggest, for example, that the patient try to speak freely and openly while the therapist listens and makes whatever comments might be helpful. Such a proposal certainly sounds reasonable and potentially helpful. It defines both the therapist's and the patient's role in a clear although limited fashion. It does not, however, say anything about what the patient is to do with the therapist's "helpful comments." The therapist may think the patient already understands what to do, or indeed may think the patient should *not* be told what to. In either event, the patient may not know what the therapist thinks the patient knows, so that both the therapist's comments and the patient's responses lead only to confusion. Of more concern in this example of a limited agreement is that it says nothing about the purpose of proceeding in this manner. The therapist's passivity and sparse verbal responses may or may not help the patient get where he or she hopes to go. The therapist and patient have not agreed on where that should be or on whether the therapy style proposed is the best way to get there. As a result, if the patient benefits, it will be only because of the accidental match between what is employed and what will work best. We ought to be better able to provide effective therapy than by a reliance on mere luck.

A false agreement is even more destructive. Suppose the patient signs on to the above proposal for an unstructured and open-ended therapeutic style but really wants some specific and limited advice. As the string of sessions progresses, and no advice is forthcoming, the patient will feel increasingly frustrated and may drop out of treatment. At best, he or she may finally communicate this frustration to the therapist, who will perhaps offer some helpful comments about the difficulties appearing in their relationship and ask the patient to consider whether they come from earlier relationships. Even an invitation to explore the transference, however, misses the point that the patient's frustration is justified. It is as if one went to a lawyer to have a will drawn up and was presented instead with a title search on one's property. Such a mismatch of expectations and results may be unlikely in law practices but unfortunately not in psychotherapy offices.

To avoid such a false agreement, the therapist must make it clear what he or she proposes to do and ask the patient if the proposal matches the patient's expectations. With discussion and negotiation, they may reach agreement on the *process* of therapy to be followed. At this point, they have avoided a false agreement, but they still face an incomplete agreement because they have not agreed on *why* they are using this particular approach. In other words, having agreed on the STRATEGY, their therapeutic contract will not be complete unless they also agree on the AIM of their work and the GOALS that are expected to bring it about.

Absent or Incomplete Aim

When therapy begins without a decision about the best possible outcome or when the AIM selected is itself a poor choice, the therapy flounders haphazardly or is guided by the random choice of a series of interesting but irrelevant GOALS. When the AIM represents only some of the therapist's hopes or only part of the patient's expectations, the initial progress of therapy may last longer. Therapist and patient covertly disagree, but it will take some time for the disagreement to emerge. Sooner or later the therapy will be so far off the expectation of either that effort and energy will be expended in a diffuse and unproductive way. As this happens, progress will slow and finally stop.

Poor Selection of Goals

A poorly chosen GOAL may lead the therapy to a structural impasse in three ways. First, the problem GOAL might be unrealistic or represent more than therapy can accomplish. Therapy cannot, for example, overcome a bad social system or create helpful changes in a family member who declines to join the session. Other GOALS ask for more than the patient can achieve. Trying to help a patient to become more intelligent, for example, or to overcome long-standing impulsivity, or to develop empathy where none has existed may fit the old adage about turning a sow's ear into a silk purse. Unrealistic GOALS lead to wasted effort and frustration. Second, the GOAL might be unrelated to the overall purpose of the therapy. Although the GOAL may be reasonable on its own merits and even desirable, it may have nothing to do with the matters at hand. For example, a therapy that hopes to ameliorate a marital problem but concentrates on a GOAL of helping the patient overcome job difficulties may end up accomplishing neither. Even when achieved, an unrelated GOAL will not advance the therapy as a whole because it will not contribute to the AIM. Third, the GOAL might have negative effects. It might, for example, stir up overwhelming anxiety and activate a psychotic process. It might instead stimulate such an intense reaction outside of therapy as to threaten the patient's family or social status. Ameliorating the guilt over an old infidelity, for instance, might provoke an unnecessary confession, upset the spouse, and cause the couple to separate. Developing more assertiveness in an employee could prove so disruptive in the workplace that it would undermine the patient's job security. The unwitting pursuit of a GOAL with potentially negative consequences will threaten the continuity of the therapy.

Yet if other therapy GOALS are realistic and relevant and have positive effects, the one problem GOAL can usually be revised or modified. In the examples given above, GOALS might be reworked to make better use of whatever intelligence level or empathic ability the patient possesses, the job difficulties can be deferred as a later piece of therapy planning, the guilt over infidelity can be reframed from a marital issue to a values issue, and assertiveness training can be redirected into a safer area of experience. The overall course of the therapy can then continue in line with the original plan.

RESOLVING THE STRUCTURAL IMPASSE

The first requirement in resolving a structural impasse is to recognize that one exists. If therapist and patient have not built a plan together, they will have no basis for this recognition. They may try one remedy after another in an effort to resolve the impasse, all without result, and recognize that the treatment plan is the source of the problem only when other explanations fail. A positive recognition of the impasse, based on their earlier work of constructing the treatment plan, serves them better than finding the answer through a process of exclusion.

Unplanned therapy may nevertheless have a structure. The structure may be imposed by the methodology, as would be the case in classical psychoanalysis, or by the therapist's habit of approaching cases in routine ways. An example of the latter is a desensitization protocol. This unplanned structure may not fit the patient's needs. It may ignore the patient's requests in favor of the therapist's preferences. It may be the wrong structure for the particular patient. When this unplanned structure fails to meet the patient's needs and an impasse results, the therapist may not recognize the source of the problem.

Early recognition of a structural impasse is more likely if the therapist remains alert to it—in other words, if the therapist has what is customarily called a high index of suspicion. The use of treatment planning as a deliberate step in consultation and in the initiation of treatment trains the therapist to think of treatment plan difficulties as soon as an impasse begins to develop. Signposts and benchmarks, recommended as a way of tracking the progress of a plan, are useful signals of a potential impasse when they fail to appear as expected. Periodic review of the treatment plan, useful enough in keeping therapy focused and moving forward, will call the therapist's attention to any of those areas whose lagging progress will flag an evolving impasse. The practice of writing out the treatment plan, keeping it as a part of the patient's clinical record, and referring to it regularly as the work proceeds will increase the likelihood that an impasse will be recognized early.

Once recognized, a structural impasse is corrected by the same process used to create the original plan: assessment, formulation, planning, and negotiation. If therapy got under way without a treatment plan—a common precedent to an impasse—the process can start from there. In effect, the therapist initiates a fresh consultation period, and the patient must be made aware of the new effort. Patients often know when therapy is not going well and generally respond favorably to a new start. The therapist can suggest that they sit back and take another look at what they are doing and what they want to do from this point forward. Solving the impasse when the issue is the entire plan may depend on one or more of the essential steps. The key element may be the thoroughness of the assessment or it may be the accuracy of the formulation. Once assured that these two elements have been adequately addressed, the therapist can move ahead to the plan itself. As usual, the indispensable follow-up step to the therapist's plan is sharing the ideas with the patient, clarifying the patient's requests, and bringing them together in a form acceptable to both parties.

If the impasse is traceable to an inaccurate AIM or arises from problems with any of the GOALS, a less extensive correction will suffice. Perhaps the formulation must be reexamined to restate the AIM in a more useful way. Perhaps the agreement with the patient concealed some uncertainties or hesitations that rendered it less than genuine. Unrealistic GOALS can be modified to more attainable objectives. Negative GOALS can be reframed to be less threatening, or they can be abandoned altogether.

Not every structural impasse is correctable. On occasion, the tensions it engenders are too threatening to allow the patient to remain in a working alliance with the therapist. At the other extreme, it may turn out, on investigating the source of the impasse, that the patient does not require psychotherapy as first appeared. Sometimes patients present with problems or requests that are not suitable for psychotherapy and must be referred elsewhere. It is even possible that on second look, the patient is doing well enough already.

Another reason for an irresolvable impasse is the inability to reach an agreement. Sometimes no amount of negotiation can bridge the gap between what the patient wants and what the therapist is prepared to attempt. The reasons for such a mismatch are multiple, but common issues include the therapist's requirement of a therapeutic approach the patient finds unacceptable, the patient's insistence on boundary violations the therapist is unwilling to grant, and other relationship issues. An intractable disagreement can arise over the nature of the problem itself, especially with patients whose reality testing is impaired or whose personalities are excessively rigid. Sometimes time and money issues cannot be reconciled. Occasionally the issue is one over which neither has control, such as gender or age.

Unless the patient has dropped out of treatment and thereby made any question of negotiation moot, most structural impasses can be resolved, and the treatment process is the stronger for it. Irresolvable impasses, when they do occur, require that the patient be given the therapist's best advice and allowed to leave. Hopefully, such a patient will accept a referral to another practitioner.

Chapter 12

PLANNING WITH "DIFFICULT" PATIENTS

Successful treatment planning, as I have described it, requires certain accommodating but variable patient characteristics. The ability to form a working alliance, the intelligence to understand the issues involved in planning, and the flexibility to participate in the give-and-take of negotiation all favor successful planning. Impaired reality testing, the inability to deal honestly with the therapist, and overwhelming external stresses will militate against that success. Patients falling within certain diagnostic groups are likely to have difficulties with one or more of these characteristics. In reviewing these groups, I highlight problem areas that other patients will also present in a more elusive manner. The less obvious presentation of these problems will make recognition more difficult and therefore resolution harder. The therapist who learns to identify these problems when more sharply delineated will find them easier to recognize in more subtle presentations.

COGNITIVE IMPAIRMENT

Patients with borderline or low intelligence, and those who present with developmental or neurological deficits that impair abstraction and other cognitive abilities, will have difficulty understanding the process of treatment planning as well as the concepts underlying it. These deficits occur not only with mentally retarded patients, developmentally disabled patients, and those with dementia but also in patients with chronic psychoses and secondary neurological impairments. Therapy with these patients must often settle for more limited aspirations than for those with a normal or intact brain. Nevertheless, to the extent that psychotherapy is a useful part of their overall treatment, a clear and acceptable treatment plan will be helpful in working with these patients. The therapist must adapt the plan to the recognized deficits and compromise on a more circumscribed therapy result.

ADDICTION

Addicted individuals have a problem with the contractual aspect of treatment planning. They may have difficulty entering into the working alliance because of the conflict between embracing the treatment and giving up the addiction on the one hand and sabotaging the treatment and continuing the addiction on the other. Where addictive problems are joined with poor impulse control, the patient may have trouble not only reaching an agreement but also sticking to it.

Working with these patients is one of the treatment situations in which the process of negotiation is itself of potential therapeutic benefit. Success in dealing honestly with the therapist pays off not only in the higher likelihood of maintaining abstinence but also in the possibility that that success will generalize to other significant relationships as well.

It is especially important with addicted patients to be sure of agreement on the desired outcome of the therapy. The therapist may feel that abstinence is the only logical AIM, whereas the patient may want to find a way to continue the pleasures of the addiction without suffering its negative consequences. Resolution of this common disagreement may take a good deal of work.

PSYCHOSIS

Psychotic patients are likely to disagree with the therapist on the nature and the priorities of the problems. The therapist might consider the primary issue to be management of the psychotic disorganization and of the potential risks to the patient or others. The patient may want help in dealing with enemies that are products of his or her delusions or want support for pathological relationships with employers or family members. If agreement is not reached on the problems presented, deciding on treatment GOALS is equally complicated. High levels of anxiety, significant mood disturbances, and the reality of impairment itself may make it difficult to preserve the rational foundation of a working alliance. There may be similar difficulties in reaching agreement on treatment STRATEGIES, as, for example, the need for medication to stabilize a patient with a paranoid psychosis.

In outpatient settings, chronically psychotic patients may present with relatively stable, albeit low, levels of recovery. Realistic assessment may suggest that treatment GOALS be limited. The therapist might only want to help the person remain stable enough to prevent another hospitalization. Important as these GOALS are, individual psychotherapy may not represent the central part of the treatment effort.

CHARACTER PATHOLOGY

In treating people with personality disorders, the planning process meets challenges at several levels.

Determining the AIM is often difficult. Personality difficulties shade from the disabling state of a full-blown disorder through degrees of more-or-less troublesome trait disturbances and into the blurry border of normality. Pervasive but ego-syntonic behaviors may or may not cause subjective distress. The therapist is tempted to define the AIM in abstract terms that are difficult to translate into meaningful treatment GOALS. *Emotional independence*, *stable relationships*, and *trust* are examples. It is more useful, however, to propose something more concrete to the patient as the hoped-for outcome of therapy. *Emotional self-sufficiency within the family* might be doable. *A stable marriage relationship* could be at least a beginning definition. *Trustfulness in peer relationships* would be worth discussing.

Treatment GOALS may also resist definition. If the AIM is abstractly vague, the therapeutic objectives that will realize it become hard to specify, and therapists may feel they are building on a foundation of sand. As an alternative, therapists may feel tempted to base the GOALS on the patients' complaints rather than their requests. Thus, a man who complains of persecution by his employer might be told therapy will explore why he is especially sensitive to the situation. This solution substitutes a process for a result—in other words, a STRATEGY for a GOAL. What, then, should the GOAL be? A job change? Assertiveness? Diminished use of projective identification? Without a clearly delineated AIM, there is little basis for rational choice.

As these distinctions show, however, the tension between planned and unplanned therapy is strongest in regard to patients whose primary diagnosis is a personality disorder. These patients are often selected for expressive therapies with a reconstructive rationale and a long-term orientation. Almost by design, such an approach eschews a stipulated result and plans to follow wherever the patient might lead. Issues of transference, symptomatic behavior, and acting out lend weight to this design. A patient offered this approach may accept the indeterminate nature of the treatment, so that a therapeutic contract is reached without specified terms. Under these conditions, therapy is truly open ended. Neither patient nor therapist has a solid basis for recognizing when therapy has succeeded. Neither can tell, therefore, when it is over. These therapies are most at risk for becoming interminable.

If therapist and patient attempt a negotiation, the effort to reach a therapeutic agreement becomes entangled with the very traits that precipitated the patient's request for help. Antisocial patients will manipulate the process instead of dealing honestly with the therapist. Dependent patients may agree, out of a need for acceptance by the therapist, with anything proposed. Obsessive patients may view the contracting process as a struggle for control and adopt a legalistic, oppositional stance. Here therapists must engage patients in the same treatment process they intend for the therapy proper to get past the patients' traits and arrive at an agreement. Using the treatment process as the means to reach agreement might seem to put the cart before the horse, but this reversal is not necessarily unproductive. A good deal of work can be usefully done in the service of reaching a contract. With some patients, the negotiating process continues throughout therapy, making it the framework within which therapy functions.

SOME SPECIAL PROBLEMS WITH PATIENTS WITH BORDERLINE PERSONALITY DISORDER

Patients with borderline personality disorder present a number of treatment challenges. High on the list are 1) formulating the case to construct a useful treatment plan, 2) arriving at a reasonable and stable treatment contract, and 3) carrying the therapy through to an optimally timed termination. Any brief discussion of borderline issues will necessarily be oversimplified, but it does provide at least a point of reference for the treatment planning issues that concern us here.

Goldstein (1990) noted the remarkable diversity in theory and practical approaches to the borderline syndrome. She divided them into two groups. The *conflict model*, propounded by Kernberg, Masterson, and others, describes this disorder as a rigid and maladaptive defensive structure that originates in childhood. This persistent defensive structure works to contain intrapsychic conflict. It requires a confrontive and interpretive therapy approach, sometimes under the controlled conditions of limit setting and an externally imposed structure. Therapy is generally intensive and long term. The *deficit model*, derived from the work of Hartmann, Mahler, Kohut, and others, understands borderline symptomatology as a reflection or expression of personality deficits, underdeveloped aspects of the self, of ego functions, and of object relations. Treatment endeavors to build or rebuild the missing or deficient personality structures through a flexible approach modified by the patient's individual needs. Therapists may vary the intensity and duration of therapy.

These two very different formulations lead, as might be expected, to different treatment plans. The AIM, however, is similar in both constructions. To oversimplify again, it is usually a statement emphasizing the need to promote identity integration. Stevenson and Meares (1992), for example, said that the "aim is maturational. Specifically, it is to help the patient discover, elaborate and represent a personal reality" (p. 358).

The conflict and deficit models differ more widely in the GOALS and STRATEGIES each one emphasizes. The conflict model, for example, would measure progress in therapy by the diminution of pathological defenses, such as splitting, and the improvement in existing internalized object relations. The deficit model would emphasize the growth of helpful new internalized objects and advances in self-cohesion. STRATEGIES differ as well, with the conflict-based model leaning toward a neutral, abstinent stance, and the deficit-based model tending toward a more active and selectively gratifying stance.

These various approaches show that different theoretical constructions can translate into practical treatment plans. The key to doing so, however, is the accuracy with which the formulation addresses the individual patient's specific life circumstances, needs, and expectations.

Among the consistently demanding issues presented by patients with borderline personality disorder, none is more difficult than establishing and maintaining a treatment contract. Elements of the treatment contract would include the conditions of treatment (the frequency and length of sessions, fees, the handling of telephone contacts), the nature of the relationship (patient-therapist boundaries, the therapist's activeness and degree of self-disclosure), and the nature of the problem (the AIM) and of the treatment itself (GOALS and STRATEGIES).

According to DSM-IV-TR (American Psychiatric Association 2000), a diagnosis of borderline personality disorder requires that at least five of nine criteria be met (see Table 12–1).

TABLE 12–1. Diagnostic criteria for borderline personality disorder

Five or more of the following criteria must be met for a diagnosis of borderline personality disorder:
1. Frantic efforts to avoid real or imagined abandonment
2. A pattern of unstable and intense interpersonal relationships characterized by alternating between extremes of idealization and devaluation
3. Identity disturbance: markedly and persistently unstable self-image or sense of self
4. Impulsivity in at least two areas that are potentially self-damaging
5. Recurrent suicidal or self-mutilating behavior
6. Affective instability
7. Chronic feelings of emptiness
8. Inappropriate, intense, difficult-to-control anger
9. Transient, stress-related paranoid ideation or severe dissociative symptoms

Source.   Adapted from American Psychiatric Association 2000.

The listed characteristics illuminate the difficulties in reaching agreement with these patients. Limitations on time, the therapist's availability, and other conditions of treatment intensify the patient's sensitivity to threats of abandonment. That sensitivity plus the affective instability make any discussion of limitations on time or on the availability of the therapist—the conditions of treatment—a stressful experience that can provoke disabling anxiety, dissociative or paranoid symptoms, or outbursts of rage. The patient's feeling of chronic emptiness and the difficulty with maintaining a constant, stable relationship with the therapist threaten the working alliance and disrupt the effort to define the relationship. The threat of suicidal or self-mutilating behavior creates a high-risk environment for the negotiating process. The patient's impulsivity increases the likelihood of a quick but unstable agreement on these difficult issues.

In a larger frame, the very identity disturbance that may be the core of the patient's problem makes any agreement volatile and uncertain. Who, exactly, has agreed to the treatment plan: the clinging and helpless infant, the enraged and unreasoning child, the frightened-dissociated-paranoid person, or the seemingly intact and reasonable adult? Maintaining a therapeutic alliance with a person whose mood, affect, and level of maturity seem unpredictable is perhaps the greatest challenge of all.

The sensitivity of patients with borderline personality disorder to abandonment makes termination an issue loaded with tension and potentially negative consequences. In this regard, it is interesting to consider a report (Waldinger and Gunderson 1984) that 60% of successfully treated patients with borderline personality disorder left treatment against the advice of the therapist. The therapists were highly experienced practitioners using an intensive and expressive approach. This finding suggests that therapists may not appreciate the degree of recovery in a successfully treated patient and may wish to continue the therapy longer than perhaps necessary. In a later study, Gunderson et al. (1989) noted that 36 of 60 (60%) hospitalized patients with borderline personality disorder dropped out of outpatient follow-up therapy but that "the dropouts were healthier on some baseline measures than those [patients] who continued in therapy" (p. 38). Once again, patients who left therapy before the therapist agreed to terminate might have made a greater recovery than the therapist appreciated.

The treatment plan can soften the stress of termination to some degree by making the issue overt and concrete. Therapist and patient should discuss the certainty that the treatment will end, even though the date may be uncertain. This discussion should include the patient's role in deciding when to terminate. The therapist's judgment that the treatment plan may be near its GOALS and about to achieve its AIM—that is, that termination is imminent—is likely to differ from the patient's view.

Termination should remain on the table throughout the treatment period. It can be continually reexamined and discussed so that its terrors moderate as much as possible. If the therapist keeps in mind the GOALS and AIM of treatment, therapy will not drift past the point where its maximum benefits have been achieved.

OTHER PLANNING CHALLENGES

Other issues that complicate treatment planning include long-term work, consultation, co-therapy arrangements, and third-party reviews.

Treatment Planning for Long-Term Therapy

Most psychotherapy is relatively short term. The median duration is four to eight visits; only about 10%–15% of patients continue for 20–25 visits or more (Olfson and Pincus 1994). *Long term* is a relative concept: Twenty-five weekly visits is less than 6 months of therapy. Nevertheless, the longer the therapy continues, the more difficult it is to maintain focus on the treatment plan.

Many factors conspire to diffuse the effort. Intercurrent crises divert energy and concern. Life circumstances change. Transference and countertransference issues require attention. Other resistances emerge as the exploration of designated subjects evokes anxiety and avoidance. The patient who agreed to one kind of therapy effort now wants the opposite: Behavioral plans are interrupted by memories of early childhood or relationship issues, or patients in psychodynamic psychotherapy may complain about a lack of direct advice.

The first line of defense against these diffusions is to remain focused on the treatment plan and pursue it to its conclusion. The therapist can anticipate that new data, crises, life circumstances, and resistances will arise, regardless of the particular therapy approach. The treatment plan with which therapy started is presumably the best plan that patient and therapist could devise. If possible, they should press on with that original plan, but sometimes the diversion is too great to ignore. If so, it will require attention of one of two sorts. The new issues, after a thorough discussion, may be deferred until the original plan is completed and dealt with at a later time. If the new issue cannot be ignored, the treatment plan can be revised. Whether deferral or revision seems the better course is a matter of judgment and depends on the combined wisdom of patient and therapist. The important thing is that treatment continues to follow a plan and is not distracted. When planning is forgotten while the therapy pursues the latest intriguing development, the outcome is likely to be unsatisfactory.

If an intercurrent issue can be deferred and the original plan carried through, its success will reinforce the working alliance. Patient and therapist will have more confidence in their ability to work together toward another successful outcome. They can now consider the new set of issues that arose during the earlier therapy work. The planning sequence is the same: formulation based on assessment guiding the planning process, negotiation between therapist and patient leading to a new plan. In this fashion, a series of shorter-term plans are linked together to make up a long-term plan. In addition to its clarity of purpose and its efficiency, this serial treatment approach has clear benefits in dealing with managed-care systems.

Consultation

Ideally, the treatment process begins with a period of consultation followed by a period of treatment. In practice, therapists are likely to overlap or even blend these two phases. For one thing, the introduction of anticipated treatment TACTICS may help the therapist assess the patient's ability to work within the expected therapy parameters. For another, successful interventions can support the patient's motivation for treatment by showing him or her its concrete results. Finally, the time pressures of contemporary practice may encourage the therapist to begin treatment at the earliest possible stage.

There are times, however, when the clinician is only a consultant. The conditions of the consultation are that the patient will continue with someone else and that the meeting is to provide assessment and advice. The consultant is then faced with two problems: maintaining a consultation-only role and conveying the desired advice to the patient or to the referring source—or, usually, to both—in the most helpful way.

Consultation requests may originate from patients uncertain of whether they need psychotherapy or of where to get it. Third-party payers may require consultation as a condition of authorizing treatment. Nonpsychiatric physicians may ask for an opinion about the presence of significant psychiatric illness underlying organic symptoms. These requests typically arrive before any psychotherapy has begun.

Once therapy is under way, the most common stimulus to seeking an outside opinion is the absence or breakdown of a treatment plan. Either the patient or the therapist may suggest a consultation when the therapy is stalled or when the patient is no better (or is sometimes worse) than when treatment started. The consultant may recommend ways to overcome the difficulties encountered, a new direction for the therapy, or a change of therapist.

Maintaining a clear role as a consultant calls for a certain amount of restraint. Sometimes the consulting practitioner is tempted to correct the presumed faults of the therapy by direct therapeutic intervention. This temptation should be resisted because it violates the consultation agreement; it requires the consultant to act on limited information and a brief acquaintance with the patient and runs the risk of falling into the patient's acting out or manipulative behavior toward the referring therapist; it puts the consultant in the awkward position of starting something he or she cannot finish; and it may create a conflict of interest between the role of consultant and that of therapist.

Often the most helpful advice the consultant can provide is to identify the impasse as a problem with the treatment plan. This help may include questioning the apparent AIM of the troubled therapy or the relevance of its GOALS or even the selection of treatment STRATEGIES. It may mean suggesting a treatment plan when one is not discernible in the work the patient and therapist have done so far. How this information is conveyed to both parties is sometimes a delicate exercise in diplomatic discourse, especially when the referring therapist does not share the same frame of reference as the consultant who understands the importance of treatment planning.

Co-Therapy

Working with another therapist can be a difficult undertaking, posing the challenge of managing two sets of relationships at the same time. The two therapists must not only deal with the patient with whom they are jointly working but must also maintain a productive working relationship with each other. A common arrangement is a nonmedical therapist using a psychiatrist or primary care physician as a medical consultant.

Here treatment planning may make an important contribution. The same process applies as if only one therapist was making the assessment, constructing the formulation, and translating it into AIM, GOALS, and STRATEGIES, although with both therapists contributing to it. Again, the negotiating phase must deal with the patients' requests as they inform and modify the final plan. All of these steps may be complicated by the addition of another set of ideas and preferences. The end result, the final plan, should be worth the effort.

The experience of negotiating with each other, as well as with the patients, lays a foundation for the close collaboration that nurtures a successful co-therapy association. The need to communicate with each other both in the planning and in the implementation of the therapy assists the co-therapy effort. The structured approach provided by the treatment plan helps to focus both therapists on the same issues and interventions. All of these supports should strengthen the co-therapy relationship and improve the chances for a favorable outcome.

Third-Party Review

Third parties intrude more and more into therapeutic relationships and may require a treatment plan before they will approve payment. When confronted with a reviewer to whom they must justify the proposed therapy, therapists will be in a stronger position if they can present a coherent and well-thought-out treatment plan. Although reviewers may come from a clinical background and carry the credentials of a mental health professional, they are not always sufficiently familiar with the requirements of direct clinical work. The front-line exigencies of clinical practice, in whatever setting it may occur, can create a communication barrier with the less-experienced reviewer.

Merely having a plan is at once an advantage in dealing with reviewers. Their usual encounters with therapists, particularly in outpatient psychotherapy reviews, will likely have left the impression that most psychotherapy is unplanned. Even where therapists have had a treatment plan, they may have had difficulty in communicating it to reviewers in a form that made sense to the reviewers. Thus when a therapist can say, "This is what my work with this patient ought to accomplish, and these are the steps that will bring it about, and this is the method I intend to use to take those steps," the reviewer can anticipate a reasonable chance of completing the task he or she was hired to perform. The reviewer's relief at this prospect is favorable to the therapist and to the plan the therapist wants authorized.

As indicated, the therapist may have to translate the concepts and terminology into language that the reviewer will understand. Reviewers have to deal with a variety of therapists, some of whom use unfamiliar or esoteric jargon. The reviewer may feel the therapist is talking down to a presumed inferior or is deliberately obfuscating the case to avoid scrutiny. The therapist with a plan to present can do so with confidence and clarity. In general, the more concrete and conventional the language, the more acceptable the plan is likely to be.

REFERENCES

American Psychiatric Association: Diagnostic and Statistical Manual of Mental Disorders, 4th Edition, Text Revision. Washington, DC, American Psychiatric Association, 2000

Goldstein EG: Borderline Disorders: Clinical Models and Techniques. New York, Guilford, 1990

Gunderson JG, Frank AF, Ronningstam EF, et al: Early discontinuance of borderline patients from psychotherapy. J Nerv Ment Dis 177: 38–42, 1989

Olfson M, Pincus HA: Outpatient psychotherapy in the United States, I: volume, costs, and user characteristics. Am J Psychiatry 151: 1281–1288, 1994

Stevenson J, Meares R: An outcome study of psychotherapy for patients with borderline personality disorder. Am J Psychiatry 149: 358–362, 1992

Waldinger RJ, Gunderson JG: Completed psychotherapies with borderline patients. Am J Psychiatry 38:190–201, 1984

Chapter 13

LEARNING TO PLAN TREATMENT

The use of multiple treatment modalities (STRATEGIES) in the clinical examples presented earlier might have raised some doubts about the ability of one therapist to be skilled in a variety of therapeutic approaches. Can we be both a knowledgeable and creative behavioral therapist and an insightful and skilled psychodynamic therapist and employ cognitive therapy skills at a competent level as well? Can we have both the non-intrusive approach of the empathic existentialist and the directive authority of a behavioral therapist? What is the sense of selecting different modalities to treat a patient if the therapist is not competent in more than one set of psychotherapy skills?

I believe most therapists are capable of expanding their therapeutic armamentarium, although they may impose limitations on themselves, especially if they were exposed in training to only a single approach. (That in fact was my own experience; my residency training faculty was heavily weighted with Freudian psychoanalysts who were convinced that all other approaches—behavioral, short-term, even [in some cases] medication—were useless and even unethical.) Therapists who have confidence in one type of psychotherapy, especially if it required much time and effort to acquire, may feel they cannot perform competently with an unfamiliar although promising alternative and may select patients who accommodate to their system rather than those whose problems require something different. The personality style of the therapist may also influence the choice of approach. Some will prefer a more active, interventionist therapy; others, a more reflective and laissez-faire process. Therapists (and their patients) can benefit, however, from efforts to overcome these limitations. A therapist needs a working knowledge of multiple approaches to deal successfully with the variety of patients who present themselves for treatment. Developing comfort and expertise with the widest possible range of therapeutic modalities is likely to improve any therapist's rate of success.

As you read through the brief histories presented in this book, you might have disagreed with the particular way I looked at the case. Perhaps you thought of other approaches, some simpler, others more complex, that you would have considered if you were taking care of the patient. You might have used other theoretical constructions, and even if you would have chosen the same approach, you might have disagreed with the way I presented it. This disagreement is to be expected in a profession such as ours, in which many viable lines of inquiry, from the macrobiological to the cultural, energize our field with new ideas and encourage the creative imagination to explore them to the fullest extent. There is often no one right way to understand and formulate a case, and there are, fortunately, many treatment options available to those with the knowledge and experience to use them. Success favors those who have a variety of skills, within different therapy approaches, from which they can choose the best therapy for the particular patient with whom they are working at the moment. The more carefully therapists plan for what they do, the more likely it is they will choose the best treatment and set out the best course for their patients. Planning improves psychotherapy, regardless of the approaches followed or the technical skills employed.

Treatment planning, like other aspects of psychotherapy, can be learned in two ways. The first is self-study, part of the process of continuing education that allows one to develop professionally over the course of a career. Self-study is often informal and unguided, focused on issues of varying importance, with topics selected by chance encounters with interesting material or particularly challenging patients. It may result in a hodgepodge of new learning, little of which carries through to the progressive accumulation of new expert skills. Yet properly done, self-study can be of great value. The second path of learning is through formal training. Although all of us began with this advantage, as we prepared within our professional specialty, formal training, too, can become fragmented and sporadic, driven by licensing and professional requirements rather than by relevance or genuine interest. Still, it is often an advantage to acquire new skills through a prescribed training exercise, one that offers built-in discipline and corrective feedback from an expert in the field of study. Both of these avenues can be helpful in learning how best to use treatment planning and in sharpening the skills that enhance its use.

Once therapists have completed their training, they are expected to seek out and participate in continuing education within their professional discipline. Although a great variety of educational programming and opportunity is available, relatively little of it is directly concerned with treatment planning. Of the several professional disciplines that comprise the mental health network, only psychiatric nursing places a consistent historical emphasis on treatment planning, especially with regard to psychodynamic psychotherapy (Webster et al. 1994). Where they exist, formal programs about treatment planning appear to concentrate on inpatient rather than outpatient services, and a specific program on treatment planning in psychotherapy is, so far as I can determine, a rarity. Until this topic is more readily covered through educational programming, therapists who wish to improve their planning skills will have to do so through individual and peer supervision.

Working with an experienced supervisor can be profitable throughout one's professional career. Clinicians have little opportunity to observe psychotherapy directly and must rely on personal experiences and interpersonal skills. An individual supervisor can enhance a therapist's professional growth by serving as a model, as a sounding board, and as a teacher.

Not all supervisors will be equally helpful with treatment planning. Some may be philosophically opposed to the concept itself. Others may accept the concept but neglect it in their supervisory work. Still others may not think of planning as a central issue in all psychotherapies. They may include it in reviewing a behavioral plan, for instance, but not when the approach is psychodynamic psychotherapy. It is up to the supervisee who is interested in this aspect of treatment to raise it with the supervisor. It might be useful to negotiate a supervisory plan that will make becoming skilled at treatment planning one of the educational goals. It may be necessary to remind the supervisor of your continued interest if the topic seems to drop in priority or importance.

Peer supervision is another way to learn treatment planning through a formal educational effort. Its flexibility and unofficial status make it more accessible to experienced therapists no longer attached to an institutional training program. Peer supervision groups exist in different sizes and undertake different missions. Whether the group is a stable dyad or a large and shifting aggregate of therapists, however, it must determine its agenda and process. Will it follow one case over time? A different case from each therapist every week? Will it be a free-for-all discussion? A single discussant? These and other choices may be made overtly or simply develop as the group's particular traditions.

A peer supervision group must decide whether to concentrate on treatment planning and, if so, to what extent. Not all members may be equally interested. The level of competence may vary. The group can be most helpful, in my view, by concentrating on two points in the planning process. The first point of concentration should be the formulation. Discussions of completeness and of the success with which the offered formulation explains or models the patient's overall presentation will be helpful. Emphasizing the cause-and-effect side of the formulation will be more useful than examining its descriptive side in greater detail than the therapist offers. I am concerned here with the inclination of groups of listeners to ask for more and more clinical information, no doubt to test their own (unspoken) ideas. These informational disruptions distract the discussion from its main purpose: to help the presenters manage their cases and sharpen their clinical skills. The group must understand the formulation as the foundation of treatment planning to help a group member achieve these ends. The second point of concentration should be the completed treatment plan. Copies of the written planning diagram will help group members understand the plan graphically and will facilitate review. Discussing the plan from a top-down perspective will be more useful than a random focus on one or another element, or on the strategic and tactical elements to the neglect of the AIM and GOALS. Group members must share a common understanding and vocabulary of the planning approach if the discussion is to be inclusive and meaningful.

A core element of the planning approach I have presented is the use of multiple therapeutic modalities. The implementation of a carefully prepared treatment plan will be only as successful as its component therapeutic approaches. In other terms: GOALS cannot be reached without successful STRATEGIES; successful STRATEGIES require effective TACTICS. The challenge we face as therapists is to expand our range of therapeutic skills even as we polish the skills we have already gained. Perhaps it is useful to look at the challenge in terms of a set of nested boxes (Figure 13–1). In the central box are the *core therapies*. These are the therapies in which we are most experienced and comfortable. We have the highest confidence in our ability to use these modalities to meet the widest range of therapeutic challenges from the beginning of a therapy to its end. These core modalities sit within a middle box of *adjunctive therapies*. These are therapeutic approaches with which we feel confident and have a reasonable amount of clinical experience. We tend to use these modalities when a particular clinical situation requires them. Despite our preference for one of our core therapies, we select an adjunctive approach because we believe it better fits the needs of a particular patient. The outer box contains a group of therapies in which we are developing expertise. At a later point, we expect them to become adjunctive therapies or perhaps even join the smaller number of core therapies that we use most frequently. These therapies represent *learning in progress*. Although we would not want to rely on them entirely, we may be experienced

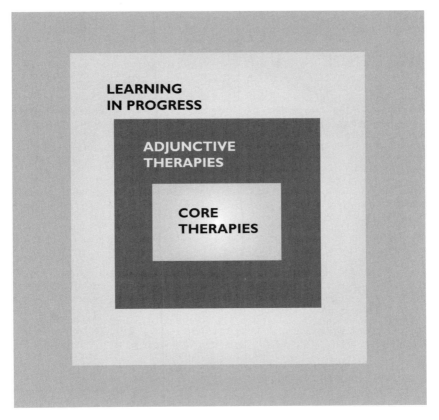

FIGURE 13–1

RANGE OF THERAPEUTIC MODALITIES

LEARNING IN PROGRESS

ADJUNCTIVE THERAPIES

CORE THERAPIES

enough with them to use them under optimum circumstances and, even better, under supervision from someone more expert in their use.

For example, a therapist might prefer to treat patients with a psychodynamic approach (that therapist's core therapy) but will instead use cognitive-behavioral therapy, an adjunctive therapy, when confronted with a patient whose overriding problem is agoraphobia. The therapist may prefer to work in individual psychotherapy but use a family systems approach when it seems indicated. A different therapist, of course, might prefer family therapy to individual therapy and a cognitive approach over a psychodynamic one and choose the same therapeutic modalities if presented with the same patient.

Continuing professional education is an effort to expand these circles of expertise. We try to add to and widen our core therapy set and to move as many therapies as possible from the learning circle to the adjunctive section. In this effort, we can use formal training and self-study, individual learning, and supervised work to grow and develop as experts in psychotherapy.

REFERENCE

Webster DC, Vaughn K, Martinez R: Introducing solution-focused approaches to staff in inpatient psychiatric settings. Arch Psychiatr Nurs 8:254–261, 1994

INDEX

Page numbers printed in **boldface** *type refer to tables or figures*